100 Questions & Answers About Coronaviruses

Delthia Ricks, MS

Author: *100 Questions & Answers About Influenza*

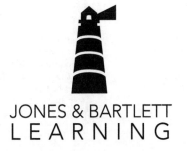

JONES & BARTLETT
LEARNING

World Headquarters
Jones & Bartlett Learning
5 Wall Street
Burlington, MA 01803
978-443-5000
info@jblearning.com
www.jblearning.com

Jones & Bartlett Learning books and products are available through most bookstores and online booksellers. To contact Jones & Bartlett Learning directly, call 800-832-0034, fax 978-443-8000, or visit our website, www.jblearning.com.

Substantial discounts on bulk quantities of Jones & Bartlett Learning publications are available to corporations, professional associations, and other qualified organizations. For details and specific discount information, contact the special sales department at Jones & Bartlett Learning via the above contact information or send an email to specialsales@jblearning.com.

Production Credits
VP, Product Development: Christine Emerton
Director of Product Management: Matt Kane
Product Manager: Joanna Gallant
Content Strategist: Melina Leon-Haley
Content Strategist: Christina Freitas
Senior Project Specialist: Dan Stone
Senior Digital Project Specialist: Angela Dooley
Marketing Manager: Lindsay White
Manufacturing and Inventory Control Supervisor: Wendy Kilborn
Composition: S4Carlisle Publishing Services
Cover Design: Scott Moden
Rights & Permissions Manager: John Rusk
Cover Image: © Alexandros Michailidis/Shutterstock
Printing and Binding: McNaughton & Gunn

ISBN: 978-1-284-22509-9

6048

Printed in the United States of America
25 24 23 22 21   10 9 8 7 6 5 4 3 2 1

CONTENTS

Part 6: Viruses 101: Superspreaders, Long Haulers, and Testing　　103

Part 7: Vaccines, Therapeutics, and Convalescent Plasma　　133

Aaron E. Glatt, MD, FACP, FIDSA, FSHEA
Chairman, Department of Medicine
Chief, Infectious Diseases & Hospital Epidemiologist
Mount Sinai South Nassau
Oceanside, NY
Professor of Medicine
Icahn School of Medicine at Mount Sinai
Mount Sinai, New York

There is essentially not a single person living in our COVID-19 world who wouldn't benefit in some way from knowing more about this devastating pandemic.

Coronaviruses have been well known and recognized as a class of very common but relatively unimportant viruses (clinically speaking) for many years. However, things changed dramatically in 2002, with the emergence of a "species-jumping" novel coronavirus that caused Severe Acute Respiratory Syndrome (aka SARS). The novel infectious agent caused very severe breathing difficulties and even death in a high percentage of infected people, and it made worldwide news on a daily basis.

SARS was a very serious infection that suddenly appeared out of nowhere and wreaked havoc throughout Asia and elsewhere in the world. Interestingly, it mysteriously disappeared, with only a brief presence between 2002 and 2004. Altogether, fewer than 10,000 people were infected, although there was a disconcerting mortality rate of approximately 10%.

Things were quiet in the coronavirus world until 2012, when another species-jumping novel coronavirus emerged, which became known as Middle Eastern Respiratory Syndrome (MERS). This disease was even more deadly than SARS, also manifesting mostly as a respiratory disease, but fortunately, it has remained restricted to a small number of people in a very limited geographic area. Unlike SARS, it still recurs every year.

However, things changed dramatically in December 2019, when the initial reports from Wuhan, China, of an illness caused by a third novel coronavirus started making medical headlines. This illness is now referred to as COVID-19: CO stands for "corona"; VI for "virus"; D for "disease"; and 19 represents 2019, the year it emerged. Initially, the new coronavirus was referred to as "the 2019 novel coronavirus" or "2019-nCoV," and in the scientific literature the virus is properly known as SARS-CoV-2 because of sequencing similarities to SARS from 2002 (which has now become SARS-CoV). *Isn't nomenclature fun?* COVID-19 has already brought forth many comparisons to the horrific 1918 influenza pandemic, which resulted in 50 to 100 million deaths, especially in many younger people. To date, there have been 94 million cases of COVID-19 worldwide, tragically with at least 2 million deaths.

That's why this marvelous book by Delthia Ricks is such an important new contribution to the understanding of the COVID-19 pandemic. Delthia has been a superb science writer for many years and has written some very significant articles and books on various infectious diseases. She brings her reporter's acumen and insight to provide us with a very readable and comprehensive book for the lay reader to realize exactly what has transpired—and what may be coming down the pike.

We remain in the midst of this life- and society-changing pandemic. The information provided in this book will hopefully be invaluable to understanding and aid in curtailing the spread of misinformation about this killer virus.

Delthia Ricks is an award-winning science journalist and author whose books include *100 Questions & Answers About Influenza*. She was a staff health and science writer for *Newsday* for 22 years where she covered a range of topics in infectious diseases, including antibiotic resistance, hospital acquired infections, and the growing threat of vaccine hesitancy. Beyond *Newsday*, she has written about novel flu viruses; the race to develop COVID-19 vaccines, and emerging gene editing technology. Her articles have been published in *Genetic Engineering and Biotechnology News, Discover Magazine,* the *Journal of the National Cancer Institute and Medical Xpress,* among other publications. Ricks' academic background is molecular and cell biology, and English literature. She holds a MS in Biology and a MA in English.

PART ONE

A Primer on Coronaviruses

What is a coronavirus? Isn't it just a
bad form of the flu?

What does the word coronavirus mean?

What are the symptoms of COVID-19?

More . . .

1. What is a coronavirus? Isn't it just a bad form of the flu?

Coronavirus

A member of the virus family Coronaviridae, which infects a wide range of animals, including mammals such as bats. Seven strains of coronavirus are known to infect humans.

Influenza

A viral respiratory illness that occurs seasonally due to strains of influenza virus from the family Orthomyxoviridae.

COVID-19

The pandemic disease initiated by a coronavirus that emerged in late 2019.

Coronavirus and flu (**influenza**) are not the same infection regardless of what self-appointed experts say. Coronaviruses belong to the vast *Coronaviridae* family, which currently includes only seven viruses known to infect humans, four of which cause relatively mild seasonal sniffles and discomforts. The virus that causes **COVID-19** and those underlying its two first cousins, SARS and MERS (see Question 6), are integral members of the same complex group of pathogens. The difference between this trio and the four that cause seasonal illnesses is that the latter three have track records of significant mortality. No member of the Coronaviridae family causes the flu because, quite simply, coronaviruses are not influenza pathogens. They belong to distinct viral families. That said, both families are respiratory viruses, meaning viral particles can be inhaled into the lungs via aerosols when a nearby infected person coughs, sneezes, or talks. Both families are members of the broad category of RNA viruses, which means their genetic material is in the form of ribonucleic acid. But those similarities pale in comparison to the substantial biological differences between the two viral families. Even though both are RNA viruses, each family arranges its genes differently inside their viral cores. Moreover, they invade different parts of human cells in the act of commandeering the host's genetic machinery. So again, despite what presidents, potentates, and armchair epidemiologists say, coronaviruses are not related to the flu.

Until the 21st century, an infection caused by a coronavirus meant a diagnosis of the common cold, and perhaps fleeting gastrointestinal symptoms. Four well-defined coronaviruses produce mild illnesses that most people treat with simple home remedies like tea and honey.

Thousands of other coronaviruses infect animals, however. Various species of bats are hosts to more than 3,200 distinct types of coronaviruses, and scientists estimate more are yet to be found. Mammals such as bats are believed to be the original hosts of the precursor coronaviruses that led to those that cause SARS, MERS, and COVID-19 (see Questions 4–6).

COVID-19 is caused by the newly identified coronavirus **SARS-CoV-2** which spawned a global **pandemic** that erupted in December of 2019. This virus, which has infected people on six of the planet's seven continents, has had such a catastrophic influence on global health and national economies that its impact is predicted to last for decades to come. It forced businesses to close worldwide, and prompted governments to enact sweeping quarantines. The World Health Organization, the agency forecasting that the pandemic's upheaval won't be easily shaken, says the planet hadn't been stricken by a global contagion as pervasive since the 1918 flu pandemic. Worse, the new viral menace has infected millions and killed hundreds of thousands of people with a vast proportion of those deaths in the United States. Sadly, more misery in terms of long-term job losses and residual pandemic-related illnesses remain on the horizon.

Influenza, on the other hand, is caused by viruses belonging to the Orthomyxoviridae family, which includes viral species that circulate seasonally among humans. Without question, the flu is a formidable infection and cannot be taken lightly: The U.S. **Centers for Disease Control and Prevention (CDC)** estimates that anywhere from 5% to 20% of the U.S. population catches the flu each year, which annually amounts to millions of coughing, achy people—and tens of thousands of deaths each year.

SARS-CoV-2
The newly identified coronavirus that causes COVID-19.

Pandemic
An outbreak of infectious disease that spreads to multiple geographic areas worldwide.

Centers for Disease Control and Prevention (CDC)
An agency of the U.S. government tasked with public health.

Both coronaviruses and influenza are capable of producing pandemics. Influenza viruses are masters of the unexpected. In 2009, a pandemic flu virus, H1N1, circled the globe; flu viruses also caused global pandemics three times in the previous century, in 1968, 1957, and most famously in 1918. Likewise, roughly once each decade in the early years of the current millennium, a coronavirus that was deemed "new to science" has set off a deadly spate of respiratory infections: SARS in 2002, MERS in 2012, and COVID-19 in 2019/2020.

2. What does the word "coronavirus" mean?

Very simply, the prefix *corona* means "crown." The term is derived from the one-dimensional appearance of a coronavirus obtained by an electron microscope more than a half century ago when these viruses were first discovered by June Almeida (see Question 3). The crown-like appearance comes from the profusion of spikes that stipple the surface of the virus. These spikes are not ornaments; they're proteins that also extend inward, deep into the virus. **Spike proteins** are vital to the pathogen as it initiates the critical event—infecting a cell.

Spike proteins
Proteins protruding from the surface of coronaviruses. In electron microscope images, these spikes impart a crown-like, or corona-like appearance, which provides the basis of name. Coronaviruses use their spikes to initiate infection. The spikes have been targeted by most developers of SARS-CoV-2 vaccines.

As previously mentioned, all coronaviruses belong to a large family of contagious agents that infect a diverse range of species from birds to mammals, including humans. Structurally, all coronaviruses have the same appearance, even though their functions are fundamentally differ ent.

A variant is any mutation—or mutations—in the DNA sequence of a prevailing virus. Mutation means change. In Britain, DNA changes in the pandemic coronavirus were detected in November 2020. The variant, dubbed B.1.1.7, became widespread throughout the United

Kingdom and by January 2021, the variant was detected globally and in multiple American states, including several with big populations, such as California, New York and Florida.

Mutations were found in the spike protein, which the virus uses to unlock human cells. The British variant is noteworthy because scientists have found that it is 50% more transmissible than its predecessor virus. In essence, it's more contagious. Despite the increased transmissibility, scientists in Britain and the United States say that doesn't mean deadlier. However, when a virus transmits more efficiently, that alone increases the number of people who potentially can become infected and wind up hospitalized, putting additional pressure on hospitals.

A variant from South Africa, detected in multiple countries, also caused coronavirus infections by early 2021. Yet another variant was reported in Japan, which was believed to have links to Brazil. While all of those variants gained notoriety, others are expected to emerge, especially in the United States. The more people transmit a virus—any virus—the more opportunities it has to mutate. Vaccines developed to provide protection against pandemic coronavirus infection are said to prevent infection by the variants.

3. When was the first coronavirus identified?

In the 1960s, teams of scientists on both sides of the Atlantic were in hot pursuit of the same goal: isolating the many viruses that cause the common cold. In 1966, virologist June Almeida emerged as a notable figure in the early days of the race. She found the first coronavirus, a pathogen that causes seasonal misery. Almeida is credited not only with identifying a common cold virus that was new to science at the time, but one with a noteworthy structure.

Identifying the first one wasn't easy. The virus was elusive and played hard to get. The sample had been taken from a sick student at a boarding school. Using an electron microscope at St. Thomas' Hospital in London, Almeida identified what seemed to be a halo encircling the virus. She and her colleagues called it a *corona*, another word for crown. The pandemic coronavirus that emerged in late 2019, SARS-CoV-2, has the same "crown" when imaged with an electron microscope. The infectious agent has a profusion of spikes. Coronaviruses, whether they cause the common cold or a deadlier infection, use the spikes to enter human cells.

4. What are the seven coronaviruses that cause human infections?

As mentioned earlier, all coronaviruses are part of the family Coronaviridae, and all are respiratory viruses. Members of this family that infect humans are also part of a subfamily called Orthocoronavirinae. Four have been known since the 1960s as causes of the common cold. Together, these four coronaviruses are believed to cause about 25% of all colds. One of those viruses, HKU1, is additionally capable of causing respiratory and gastrointestinal symptoms.

Orthocoronavirinae members are further subcategorized as either "alpha" or "beta." This type of designation determines the viral **genus**, which is based on specific molecular characteristics determined by the **International Committee on Taxonomy of Viruses (ICTV)**. The four coronaviruses associated with mild human infections are known only by numbers, letters, and genus:

Genus

With respect to viruses, the category of the coronavirus as either an alpha-or a betacoronavirus, which is determined by its specific molecular characteristics.

International Committee on Taxonomy of Viruses

An international organization created in 1966 to classify viruses and maintain a universal virus taxonomy.

- 229E (alphacoronavirus)
- NL63 (alphacoronavirus)
- OC43 (betacoronavirus)
- HKU1 (betacoronavirus)

The three viruses associated with serious disease—SARS, MERS, and COVID-19—are classified by the ICTV as betacoronaviruses, again based on genomic and molecular characteristics specified by the committee.

Each of these viruses causes a wide range of symptoms. The trio of coronaviruses that emerged in the 21st century differs from their counterparts that cause the common cold by one key factor: The newer viruses are associated with significant mortality. These viruses include:

- SARS-CoV (betacoronavirus that causes SARS)
- MERS-CoV (betacoronavirus that causes MERS)
- SARS-CoV-2 (betacoronavirus that causes COVID-19)

5. How did COVID-19 get its name?

The name "COVID-19" is simply shorthand that means **CO**rona **VI**rus **D**isease 20**19**. The year is included as an identifier to indicate when the contagion emerged. What may seem confusing is that this name is for the illness, but the virus that causes the illness has a different name: it's dubbed SARS-CoV-2.

Each name comes from different sources. The **World Health Organization (WHO)** named the *disease* COVID-19 and announced it on February 11, 2020. The *virus* was named by the ICTV, which announced its decision the same day.

World Health Organization (WHO)

The global agency, part of the United Nations, responsible for global public health.

WHO officials say it's not unusual for a disease and its causative virus to have different names. As an example, WHO's Director-General, Dr. Tedros Adhanom Ghebreyesus, cited a well-known mismatch between the names of a virus and the disease it causes: HIV, which stands for human immunodeficiency virus, is the infectious agent that causes the disease AIDS, or acquired immune deficiency syndrome.

He also defended WHO's choice of avoiding a name that was reminiscent of SARS, saying it has a negative connotation, especially in Asia, which was hard-hit by the infection in 2003.

ICTV, meanwhile, had no qualms about using SARS as part of the pathogen's name. The organization bases its naming of a virus on genetic and structural characteristics.

Members are also mindful that precise naming of a virus helps other research efforts, particularly the development of antiviral drugs and vaccines. ICTV's members are made up of virologists who describe, name, and classify every virus that infects living organisms. SARS-CoV-2's close genetic relationship to the virus that causes SARS is the reason it was given a name with the acronym SARS in it (see Question 6 for an explanation of the acronyms). However, the group did not rename SARS-CoV to SARS-CoV-1 when it announced the name for the virus that causes COVID-19.

SARS

A highly infectious disease related to COVID-19; the name is an acronym meaning **S**evere **A**cute **R**espiratory **S**yndrome.

6. What do the acronyms SARS and MERS stand for?

SARS stands for **S**evere **A**cute **R**espiratory **S**yndrome. The highly infectious disease is the closest coronavirus cousin to COVID-19.

SARS, a disease that emerged in 2002, is important in global public health history not only because it was the first explosive outbreak of the 21st century, it also was the first lethal coronavirus.

Even though the disease spread around the world, WHO did not officially declare it a pandemic. However, the CDC activated its pandemic plan to address the SARS threat as the infectious disease began its race around the world. Numerous scientific studies of the SARS era refer to this devastating episode as a global pandemic.

Although SARS infected far fewer people than COVID-19, it met the definition of a pandemic. The contagion began in the winter of 2002 in southern China. More than 8,400 people were infected in 29 countries in a wave of severe respiratory infections. Deaths numbered 744 people, according to WHO, which estimated the overall case fatality rate at roughly 10%, or 1 in 10—which is quite high when you consider that the death rate from influenza is only about 1 in 1,000. The disease was declared contained by WHO officials on July 5, 2003. After that date, the only cases of the disease were isolated laboratory outbreaks in mainland China.

Even though the SARS case fatality rate was high, it varied among the countries affected in what was clearly a pandemic. The United States recorded 27 cases, for example, and none of the patients died—so in the United States, the case fatality rate was zero. In contrast, Hong Kong, the first locality where the virus spread after the initial outbreak in mainland China, saw a case fatality rate of 17%.

SARS was particularly difficult to contain in Canada, where the case fatality rate was higher—17.1%. The contagious disease was brought into the country by air travelers from China and instantly posed extreme challenges for hospitals. The Canadian healthcare system was besieged with infections caused by a pathogen to which no one had immunity. Healthcare workers numbered prominently among Canadians who were infected. All told, there were 251 cases in Canada, and 44 deaths. Contrary to popular thinking, the SARS pandemic did not "burn itself out and go away with warmer weather." SARS was controlled through classic public health containment measures, which forced the virus out of circulation.

MERS

A coronavirus disease related to COVID-19; the name is an acronym meaning **M**iddle **E**astern **R**espiratory **S**yndrome.

MERS, meanwhile, is the acronym for Middle Eastern Respiratory Syndrome, which is caused by a virus abbreviated as MERS-CoV, or MERS-Coronavirus.

In some instances, people exposed to MERS-CoV have no symptoms, but for those who smoke or have comorbidities, such as hypertension, diabetes, or chronic lung disease, the infection can be fatal. About 35% of people who have been diagnosed with MERS died of it, according to WHO.

MERS was first identified in Saudi Arabia in 2012 and has been most frequently diagnosed among people in the Arabian Peninsula who have had direct contact with camels. Symptoms include cough, shortness of breath, and fever. Hand-washing is recommended after contact with camels. Cases have numbered under 3,000 worldwide since 2012. The MERS contagion, like SARS, has been especially lethal among healthcare workers.

7. What are the symptoms of COVID-19?

COVID-19 is a highly contagious respiratory infection that can cause a constellation of symptoms that emerge anywhere from two to 14 days after exposure. Fever, chills, cough, shortness of breath, body aches, headache, and a loss of taste and smell are key complaints.

However, according to a report in the *Annals of Internal Medicine*, a significant percentage of people exposed to the virus—40% to 45%—are asymptomatic (see Question 18) and never develop COVID-19. Even though people in this critical group don't get sick, they remain capable of transmitting the infection to others. These silent spreaders are the reason the CDC recommended wearing masks in public as the pandemic expanded in the spring of 2020. Blunting transmission became a major public health mission because people at the opposite end of the COVID-19 spectrum—those who wound up hospitalized—experienced the full brunt of a pandemic virus.

In autopsies of patients who died of COVID-19 at The Mount Sinai Hospital in New York City, Dr. Carlos Cordon-Carlo and colleagues found severe damage to the epithelium, the thin layer of cells that line blood vessels. This manifestation underlies severe blood clotting that occurs throughout the body and especially in the lungs—but no organ was spared. The clots that pervaded patients' lungs were the reason for the **hypoxia**—the low blood oxygen levels and extreme shortness of breath—that the patients experienced.

Hypoxia
Low oxygen levels in the blood.

Cordon-Carlo wasn't the only physician-scientist to witness unexpected assaults by the viral disease. A study of 5,446 COVID-19 patients treated by doctors at Northwell Health, a major New York health system, found one-third had experienced acute kidney injury. The damage was so severe many patients required dialysis. In yet another study reported in the journal *Nature*, doctors noted that because numerous organs are affected by COVID-19, the infection should be considered a multisystem disease. Dr. Aakriti Gupta of New York Presbyterian/Columbia University underscored along with her colleagues that no organ system is left unharmed. The doctors reported significant neurological problems among COVID-19 patients, which included headache, dizziness, temporary loss of the senses of taste and smell, Guillain-Barré syndrome, and, among the most severely affected, stroke. Heart problems ranged from cardiac arrhythmias to cardiogenic shock and heart attack, among several other cardiac disorders. Many COVID patients are affected by gastrointestinal disturbances, elevated liver enzymes, high blood sugar levels, and dermatologic manifestations, such as persistent rashes. In the worst of cases, patients develop the inflammatory condition known as a cytokine storm. This is a severe immune system reaction in which the body releases too many proteins known as cytokines into the bloodstream. This spurs an overwhelming inflammatory response, which leads to severe tissue injury, and even death.

The bad news didn't end there. Studies involving children hospitalized for coronavirus infection revealed that a small percentage developed a rare condition called **multisystem inflammatory syndrome in children (MIS-C)**. The disorder causes inflammation of the heart, lungs, kidneys, eyes, and brain. Before COVID-19, the syndrome didn't exist. It is most closely related to toxic shock syndrome, usually seen in bacterial infections, and Kawasaki disease, an inflammatory disorder of the blood vessels. Toxic shock syndrome is often marked by swollen hands and feet, redness of the eyes, swollen lymph nodes, and redness of the lips and tongue. Toxic shock can result in low blood pressure and fever. The CDC describes MIS-C as an extremely rare

Multisystem inflammatory syndrome in children (MIS-C)

A rare, newly identified condition associated with COVID-19 infection in children that causes inflammation of the heart, lungs, kidneys, eyes, and brain.

pediatric complication related to COVID-19. A small percentage of children with MIS-C have died of the syndrome.

8. Are some populations or ethnic groups more likely to have severe COVID-19 than others?

One of the most difficult tasks of the early pandemic era was teasing out reasons for the explosive number of deaths in the United States and why some populations fared worse than others. Nowhere in the country was high mortality more evident than in New York City, which for weeks was the nation's focal point of COVID-19. The virus swept through densely populated neighborhoods, where exposure was often inescapable. Between January and June of 2020, nearly 25,000 people died within New York State; the vast majority of those deaths were in New York City, and Black and Latino COVID-19 patients died in numbers disproportionate to their percentages in the population. Statistics from the city's Department of Health have shown that while Latinos are 29% of the city's population, they made up 34% of the COVID-19 deaths; 22% of the city's residents are Black, but they represented 28% of COVID-19's mortality.

Data from the city and state health departments also revealed that it was difficult for many in these two populations to escape the virus. Both groups had a larger proportion of **multigenerational households**, which meant if one family member was exposed in the workplace (or at school before a city-wide lockdown) the virus could be spread to multiple people at home, and especially to vulnerable grandparents. The health department's data

Multi-generational household

A household that is made up of more than two generations of related people—e.g., children, parents, and grandparents all living together.

13

further revealed that although 42% of residents are white, they accounted for 27% of the COVID-19 mortality, while Asian mortality was lowest at about 7%. Mortality tended to cluster by zip codes, a factor that led New York Governor Andrew Cuomo to establish coronavirus testing centers in COVID-19–stricken areas.

Neighborhoods that were hit hardest tended to be working-class areas where people were more likely to have jobs in so-called **essential occupations**, according to state figures. The pandemic's impact was especially evident in the working-class Wakefield neighborhood of the Bronx. Among 556 people tested there for SARS-CoV-2, 304 were positive. Census figures show the neighborhood is 58% black, 17% Latino, and 15% white.

Essential occupations

Jobs that are defined as being vital to the well-being of a community, such as grocery workers, healthcare workers, and transportation, among others.

Black and Latino residents were found to be overrepresented in several essential occupations, such as transit, grocery store, and delivery service workers. Others were employed in the healthcare industry and as emergency responders.

New York wasn't alone among states where elevated rates of COVID-19 morbidity and mortality were detected among ethnic minorities. In Texas, Florida, California, Mississippi, Alabama, and beyond, the brunt of the COVID-19 outbreak was borne by populations that were most likely to have jobs in essential occupations. As a result, COVID-19 exposed a health divide that cut along racial, ethnic, and occupational lines. Workers in the meat-packing industry throughout the Midwest, many of whom are ethnic minorities and immigrants, were sickened early in the pandemic because of close quarters and poor ventilation in meat-processing plants. Their work was declared essential by federal and state officials. In Florida, Guatemalans provide much of the labor in the state's construction industry and were among those determined to be essential workers. More than 30% of the 80,000 Guatemalan residents in the Palm Beach County area were infected early in the state's bout with SARS-CoV-2. The result, according to Florida's Department of Health, was an infection rate for Guatemalans that registered at three times the state's average.

Occupation wasn't the only driver for health disparities. In the Four Corners region of the United States, the vast Navajo Nation was so encumbered by COVID-19 that Doctors Without Borders (Medecins Sans Frontieres [MSF]) spent weeks on the reservation advising local healthcare professionals on infection control methods and aiding efforts to abate the outbreak. The Navajo Nation outbreak was determined to be among the worst in the United States. "Navajo Nation and the Pueblos people have been especially hard hit by COVID-19," Immaculata Bramlage, MSF's medical coordinator said in a statement. "Lack of access to running water and adequate infrastructure, in addition to lack of access to health care and decades of inadequate public health funding, have left people in the Navajo Nation and Pueblos extremely at-risk of contracting and suffering complications from this virus. Infection rates per capita have been some of the highest in the country."

9. Why did COVID-19 become a pandemic?

There are multiple layers to this answer, and all are of equal importance.

The virus that causes COVID-19 is noteworthy for its contagion, which is best understood in the context of it being brand new to the human population, having never circulated until its emergence in Wuhan, China, in 2019. Everyone on Earth was considered defenseless, because the human immune system had never encountered a virus like it. Although some people were infected and never developed symptoms, there remain few ways of determining who would be symptom-free once infected and who would wind up hospitalized for the infection. Public health measures that included school and business closures, travel restrictions, quarantines, and sheltering in place were aimed at casting a shield around communities to stave off infections from the novel pathogen.

Two studies from epidemiologists at Imperial College London found that shutdown orders spared lives. An estimated 60 million coronavirus infections in the United States were prevented by the measures, and 285 million were prevented in China, according to the research.

The second study found that shutdowns saved the lives of 3.1 million Europeans in 11 countries. Because of the measures undertaken in Europe, the infection rate was reduced by 82%. Still, tens of thousands of people have died, and millions were infected.

Another reason for the high rates of global morbidity and mortality are anchored in a simple fact: The coronavirus is a respiratory pathogen, which spreads easily from person to person. As unimaginable as it may seem, benign episodes of human contact helped efficiently spread the virus around the world. Respiratory droplets containing viral particles transmitted the infectious disease through simple forms of human interaction: chatting, hugging, shaking hands, or singing in a church choir. Travelers carried it across borders and time zones to every continent (including Antartica).

10. *Are there any other reasons to explain why COVID-19 became a pandemic?*

Another factor, a molecular one, underlies why COVID-19 became a pandemic: The virus has a potent affinity for a specific human protein called the **ACE2 receptor** on the surface of cells. This protein is found throughout the respiratory system, in the gastrointestinal tract, the heart and arteries, kidneys, and the eyes. The acronym ACE2 stands for *angiotensin-converting enzyme 2*. There are six other ACE enzymes, but ACE2, which additionally plays a role in blood pressure, is the one preferred by the virus that causes COVID-19.

ACE2 receptor
A protein found on the surface of cells in the respiratory system, gastrointestinal tract, circulatory system, kidneys, and eyes.

Up close in its three-dimensional form, the novel coronavirus—like all coronaviruses—roughly resembles a tiny medieval morningstar—the metal ball with spikes that 14th-century warriors wielded on a chain as a weapon. The virus infects cells by using a spike to latch onto a tiny ACE2 receptor, which protrudes from the surface of cells.

The spike binds to the receptor and in so doing converts ACE2 into a gateway. Once the coronavirus is inside the inner sanctum of the cell, the pathogen commandeers the host's genetic machinery and produces countless copies of itself. From that point, a profusion of new viruses burst free and repeat the process in nearby and distant cells. While the coronavirus that causes MERS hijacks a different receptor on human cells, the virus that causes SARS also seizes the ACE2 receptor to enter cells.

It is important to note two key differences between SARS-CoV-2 and influenza viruses. Flu viruses not only hijack human cells by unlocking a different receptor, influenza's viral RNA breaches the cell nucleus (site of the host's genes) where it replicates. SARS-CoV-2's genetic payload, a single strand of RNA, utilizes a cell's endoplasmic reticulum and Golgi apparatus to reproduce countless viral components that self-assemble into active viruses. The destructive replication process for both types of viruses destroys the cell.

11. What role do droplets play in the transmission of COVID-19 and other respiratory viruses?

Respiratory droplets

Tiny fluid particles that are suspended in exhaled air or expelled by coughing and sneezing. These particles can carry viral particles from one person to another.

Scientists who study the dynamics of viral disease transmission have examined the physiological mechanics of coughing, sneezing, talking, singing, and other vocalizations that involve the expulsion of **respiratory droplets**. Without getting too deep into the physics and mathematics of the human cough reflex, a single cough can launch virus-laden secretions at 50 miles per hour, expelling close to 3,000 respiratory droplets. Coughing has long been recognized as a key vector of respiratory infections. A sneeze is even more powerful, forcing 100,000 droplets into the immediate environment at a speed of 100 miles per hour.

These data have been collected by the American Lung Association to explain the basic physics underlying respiratory "sprays" and how they are calculated. Studies have shown that sprays can be propelled a minimum of six feet, but a growing body of evidence suggests sprays, also known as aerosols, can be propelled much farther. A flurry of studies at the Massachusetts Institute of

Technology (MIT), Texas A&M, and the California Institute of Technology have explored fine aerosols that are expelled during coughs. Droplets land on nearby objects, on one's own clothing, and the clothing of others. Infinitesimal droplets can persist in the air and be inhaled by someone within range.

Dr. Erin Bromage, a professor of comparative immunology and biology at the University of Massachusetts, Dartmouth, further estimated how exposure to respiratory droplets can drive a global pandemic. "If a person is infected, the droplets in a single cough or sneeze may contain as many as 200,000,000 (two hundred million) virus particles that can be released into the environment around them," Bromage wrote in a blog post. Although firm data on the precise number of viral particles required to cause COVID-19 remain unsettled as of this writing, Bromage—and many other researchers—theorizes that it is relatively low, amounting to approximately 1,000 particles.

Aside from coughing and sneezing, conversation between people who are only inches apart is another mode of viral transmission and another reason public health agencies stress physical distancing as a way to prevent infection with respiratory viruses of all kinds. Studies involving flu transmission have cited cigarette smoke as a method of viral infection.

Singing also expels droplets into the air space of people nearby. Several choir members in Washington State were infected with SARS-CoV-2 when one asymptomatic carrier infected most of the other singers in the group. "Singing, to a greater degree than talking, aerosolizes respiratory droplets extraordinarily well," Bromage noted.

12. Do face masks really work as a public health measure? Do they help control the spread of a pandemic virus?

The answer is yes: Wearing masks works to help control the spread of coronavirus. This isn't just true in the current pandemic: Mask-wearing, along with other nonpharmaceutical measures, helped bring an end to the SARS pandemic in the early 2000s. Countries such as New Zealand and South Korea that recommended nationwide mask usage in the COVID-19 pandemic slowed their rates of infection and contained transmission sooner. Researchers have credited Germany's face mask recommendations—and strong compliance among large swaths of the population—with helping the nation fare better in the COVID-19 pandemic than many other European countries. In Germany, face masks worked in combination with other measures—extensive antibody testing of the population and quarantining infected people—to harness viral spread. Researchers who have studied the country's use of masks concluded that facial coverings lowered the number of people who could have become infected by the virus. A study by investigators at IZA Institute of Labor Economics (Forschungsinstitut zur Zukunft der Arbeit) praised the city of Jena in the central region of the country for the local government's early recommendation that residents should wear masks. Jena boasted an especially compliant population. "After face masks were introduced on 6 April 2020, the number of new infections fell almost to zero," wrote Klaus Walde, lead author of the report. Walde and his colleagues reported strong statistical support for the use of face masks. They studied mask usage in 401 areas of Germany and concluded that while compliance differed from one area to the next, masks reduced the daily growth of infections by 40%.

In the United States, however, the CDC at first downplayed the use of face coverings but then reconsidered and recommended them. The pro-mask guidance came weeks into the pandemic after evidence of asymptomatic and presymptomatic viral spread emerged. Masks are especially recommended in areas of high transmission. Facial coverings can reduce the release of droplets into the environment during coughing, sneezing, and conversation. As the pandemic grew, the CDC took the unusual step of providing instructions on its website demonstrating how to craft a homemade mask without having to know how to sew.

CDC officials wrote in their guidance to the public that facial coverings should be used when other measures, such social distancing, are difficult to maintain. They cited grocery shopping and other essential activities as times when 6 feet of separation from others might be difficult. Masks are not for everyone, however, according to CDC guidelines. They should not be put on anyone under age two, or anyone who is unconscious, has trouble breathing, or is unable to remove the mask independently.

Dr. Lydia Bourouiba, an associate professor at MIT who has researched the biophysics of droplet movement, has found that coughing propels these secretions farther than standardized calculations suggested in years past. Bourouiba leads studies in this arcane but vital body of research at The Fluid Dynamics of Disease Laboratory, which is part of MIT. There, she and her colleagues have found that coughs and sneezes expel gaseous clouds that can travel up to 27 feet. Conducting this kind of research has relevance for epidemic and pandemic planning. Because Bourouiba has discovered that secretions travel farther than previously thought, her findings provide support for the use of masks in public.

She has captured images of test subjects sneezing and releasing massive gas clouds of secretions. "Given various combinations of an individual patient's physiology and environmental conditions, such as humidity and temperature, the gas cloud and its payload of pathogen-bearing droplets of all sizes can travel 23 to 27 feet," she wrote in the *Journal of the American Medical Association*. Bourouiba has found that droplets are propelled over great distances in a matter of seconds. "Droplets that settle along the trajectory can contaminate surfaces, while the rest remain trapped and clustered in the moving cloud," Bourouiba wrote. "Eventually the cloud and its droplet payload lose momentum and coherence, and the remaining droplets within the cloud evaporate."

In addition to the CDC, major health and medical institutions, such as the Mayo Clinic and the Johns Hopkins University Bloomberg School of Public Health, noted that mask use, frequent hand-washing, and social distancing can help prevent infection. Mask use in public was recommended by many U.S. state health departments, especially those in the Northeast, but many other states in the South, Midwest, and Southwest did not recommend the use of masks. Myths and misconceptions about mask use have unfortunately run rampant on social media (see Question 17).

PART TWO

Dispelling Myths and Misconceptions

How do we know this coronavirus came from a bat?
Is it possible that COVID-19 was made in a lab?

Can cats or dogs spread COVID-19 virus to people?

More . . .

13. How do we know this coronavirus came from a bat? Is it possible that COVID-19 was made in a lab?

Conspiracy theorists have suggested that SARS-CoV-2 was engineered at Wuhan Institute for Virology and possibly released accidentally. Yet hundreds of scientists around the world have studied and dissected SARS-CoV-2 and none have detected the telltale characteristics of genetic manipulation. They have found genetic lineage to bats, animals that are well known reservoirs of coronaviruses. Indeed, the two other deadly coronavirus diseases, SARS and MERS, also have ancestral relationships to bat coronaviruses. Despite those inescapable facts, conspiracy theories have flourished. Studies have shown that as many as one-third of Americans believe conspiracy theories about the coronavirus and its spread, including the theory that 5G mobile technology played a role in causing the pandemic.

Psychologists who have studied the pandemic say tall tales tend to surface in the midst of trauma and uncertainty. They have underscored that unusual stories—and beliefs—help people grasp difficult events. Conspiracy theories aren't new. They circulated during the 1918 pandemic when possibly as many as 100 million people died worldwide. A theory in the United States at the time blamed the Germans for creating a deadly illness and unleashing it into the world. In the COVID-19 pandemic, Donald Trump was an early proponent of the theory that the Wuhan Institute of Virology played a role in the release and spread of SARS-CoV-2. Journalist Jon Cohen, a writer for *Science* magazine, interviewed Dr. Shi Zhengli, director of the coronavirus laboratory at the Wuhan Institute. She is quoted in a July 2020 issue of the publication saying she was unaware of the new virus until samples from infected hospitalized patients were sent to her laboratory for analysis in late 2019. "Before that, we had never been in contact with or studied this virus, nor did we know of its existence," she told Cohen. Zhengli, whose nickname is Batwoman, is well known to American scientists with whom she has collaborated for decades. Zhengli is credited with leading the team of scientists who linked a bat virus to SARS.

All three serious coronavirus diseases, COVID-19, MERS and SARS are **zoonotic infections**—"spillover" viruses that have jumped from animals to people. It's unfortunate that anyone committed to the idea of a manufactured virus will probably not be open to a discussion on zoonotic diseases, infections that are caused by animal pathogens that have crossed the species barrier to infect people. Deforestation, climate change, factory farming, poaching, animal-based folk medicines, and bushmeat preparation (the killing and preparation of wild animals for food) are activities that inadvertently introduce animal pathogens to human populations.

Zoonotic infections

Infectious agents caused by animal pathogens that have jumped the species barrier to infect people.

Zoonotic viruses comprise an explosive number of emerging infectious diseases, which WHO estimates have been increasing at an alarming rate in recent decades. Bats, as it turns out, are a contributing source of viruses of all kinds—not just coronaviruses—that cause serious human diseases. Ebola and Marburg are two distinct hemorrhagic fever diseases, and both are caused by viruses belonging to the Filoviridae family. The origins of each virus can be traced to the reservoir of pathogens harbored by bats. These mammals also contributed genes to the Hendra virus, which causes a rare and deadly zoonotic disease in horses that can be passed to humans. Fruit bats in India harbor Nipah virus, which infects humans who consume fruit contaminated by bats. The disease can be lethal.

Bats don't get sick from these viruses because the viruses they host are not **pathogenic** to them—they're part of the bats' natural microbiome, just as the vast range of microbial species that inhabit the human gut don't make us sick.

Pathogenic

Causing disease.

In the June 2020 issue of the journal *Clinical Microbiology and Infection*, Dr. Nicola Petrosillo of the Lazzaro Spallanzani National Institute of Infectious Diseases in Rome reports that bat coronaviruses did not jump directly to people to cause SARS, MERS, or COVID-19.

In each instance, an intermediary animal contributed genetic material to the virus. The intermediaries involved in SARS and MERS are known; palm civets, which are short-legged, furry carnivores, are believed to have contributed genes to the virus that causes SARS. Camels contributed genes to the virus associated with MERS. Petrosillo writes that the intermediary animal involved in COVID-19 remains elusive.

As far as manufacturing it in a lab is concerned, it is far harder to prove that something *didn't* happen than it is to prove that it *did*. Scientists have plenty of evidence that these transformations happen naturally, and virologists who study coronaviruses have warned for years of the possibility for another lethal coronavirus to emerge in humans. This means that the simplest and most obvious explanation—that COVID-19 is just the latest emerging zoonotic coronavirus infection—is the most likely to be true. On the other hand, creating a brand-new, deadly viral menace in a laboratory is no easy task even for highly skilled specialists, and the precautions that would be taken in working with an infectious disease make an accidental escape—the stuff of movie thrillers and Stephen King novels—extremely unlikely. But without evidence that such an event actually occurred, it neither makes sense to speculate about it, nor does it help solve the problem at hand.

14. Do all pandemic viruses originate in China?

No. China is not the source of all pandemic viruses. The 2009 flu pandemic strain is believed to have emerged on an American-owned hog farm in Mexico; the 1918 pandemic flu virus is theorized to have roots in Kansas, although some scientific historians have argued in favor of an origin in France. The key concern related to China has been its so-called **wet markets** where fresh vegetables, butchered meats and wild, exotic animal parts have been sold. While the country's leaders have vowed to banish these markets, there have been strong associations between these venues and the emergence of serious infectious agents. SARSCoV, the virus that caused SARS in 2002, and SARS-CoV-2, which causes COVID-19, are purported to have emerged from wet markets. But these aren't the only potential viral cauldrons in China.

Wet markets
A marketplace composed of stalls that sell fresh meat, vegetables, and other perishable goods.

Yet for all the concerns about China's meat markets, there's reason for concern right here in the United States. Like dozens of other countries, the United States raises animals for their meat on factory farms. With thousands or even tens of thousands of chickens, hogs, or cattle packed into close quarters, these enterprises run the risk of becoming sources of viruses that can pass into human populations. H1N1 influenza, which traveled

Triple reassortment virus

A virus such as H1N1 influenza that has genes from three different sources. In the case of H1N1, the virus had swine, bird, and human flu genes.

around the world as a pandemic in 2009, was caused by a **triple reassortment virus**, which means it had three genetic parents—it carried swine, bird, and human flu genes. Like the virus that causes COVID-19, it was a novel pathogen. It is believed to have been harbored by swine on what was then an American-owned factory farm in central Mexico. Triple reassortment virus

Scientists worldwide are advocating for changes in how people deal with animals. Kate Jones, chair of ecology and biodiversity at University College of London, was quoted in *The Washington Post* calling for a more humane relationship with other species.

"There needs to be a cultural shift from a community level up about how we treat animals, our understanding of the dangers and biosecurity risks that we're exposing ourselves to," said Jones. "That means leaving ecosystems intact, not destroying them. It means thinking in a more long-term way."

15. Can cats or dogs spread COVID-19 virus to people?

Reports of people euthanizing pets or surrendering them to shelters due to fear of COVID-19 are heartbreaking, because there's absolutely no evidence that humans are at any risk of getting the infection from a pet. The risk of animals spreading the virus to people is considered to be low, according to a report by the CDC, and there is no evidence of animal fur carrying the virus. Because an animal's fur (or skin) cannot harbor the virus, the CDC has emphasized that pet owners should not wash their pets with harsh chemicals in a misguided attempt to "sterilize" their fur. Health officials list alcohol, hydrogen peroxide, and other disinfectants as products to avoid because they are not approved for animal use. Even though bleach was not listed by the CDC, pet owners should not use diluted or undiluted bleach on pets because it may be harmful, even deadly, to the animal.

A list of pandemic safety guidelines from the CDC advises cat owners to keep their animals indoors as much as possible and avoid allowing them to roam freely outdoors. Dogs should be walked on a leash at least 6 feet away from others, according to the guidelines.

There is, however, a small but compelling body of evidence demonstrating that people can transmit coronavirus infections to domestic and wild animals.

For example, the CDC has documented instances of human coronavirus transmission to domestic cats and dogs, but there's no evidence yet that the infection can go the other way, from the pets to their owners. Prevailing scientific wisdom based on current scientific evidence suggests that dogs are less likely than cats to become infected with the virus. This is in part because eight big cats—lions and tigers—were infected at the Bronx Zoo in New York in the spring of 2020. The animals were exposed to a human handler who was found to be an asymptomatic carrier of the virus. The felines' infections were confirmed by the United States Department of Agriculture (USDA) National Veterinary Services Laboratory in Ames, Iowa. The big cats developed a chronic cough, similar to the human reaction to coronavirus infection. Among the infected animals were Nadia, a 4-year-old female Malayan tiger, and her sister Azul. All of the animals, lions included, developed a dry cough, according to veterinarians at the zoo.

In the Netherlands, 10,000 minks that were being bred for their fur were ordered killed by farm owners after COVID-19 spread like wildfire through Dutch farming facilities. The minks caught the infection from human handlers.

Other animals known to develop infections after coronavirus exposure include ferrets and golden Syrian hamsters. The latter have been experimentally infected and are capable of spreading the virus to animals of the same species in lab settings. Pigs, chickens, and ducks are apparently immune to the virus based on limited testing and a small number of scientific research papers that were available as of this writing.

16. What is hydroxychloroquine? Is it effective against COVID-19?

Hydroxychloroquine

An antimalarial drug that is also used in treating autoimmune disorders.

Hydroxychloroquine became a target of controversy at a time when it didn't have to be in the spotlight at all. The drug has been around for decades; it's an antimalarial agent that has become a mainstay medication for people with autoimmune disorders, such as lupus. But word-of-mouth anecdotes out of China early in their coronavirus fight implied that hydroxychloroquine might hold the key to successfully treating patients with COVID-19. Subsequent research in China and France produced no solid evidence supporting this suggestion.

But that didn't stop the president of the United States from promoting it. President Donald J. Trump claimed that he successfully took the medication for two weeks. He also declared the drug "a game changer." Based largely on his promotion, millions of doses were purchased for the U.S. Strategic National Stockpile, creating shortages for patients with autoimmune disorders. The U.S. Food and Drug Administration approved it for emergency COVID-19 use, and it became the darling of Fox News—a factor that thrust the medication into a culture war. Then, problems began emerging on the scientific front. Although several studies were published highlighting hydroxychloroquine's capacity to cause heart rhythm disturbances in some patients, a major study published in *The Lancet* had to be retracted. Although *The Lancet* study also found problems among COVID-19 patients, there were concerns with the study itself. Published May 22, 2020, the research examined hydroxychloroquine and a similar drug, chloroquine and their use for COVID-19. Data in the study, however, could not be verified by independent auditors. Statistics for the research were provided by an Illinois-based analytics company, Surgisphere Corporation.

The Lancet retracted the study in June of 2020 because of the data mishap. That same month, the *New England Journal of Medicine* also retracted a COVID-19 study about heart drugs, including ACE2 inhibitors, citing unverifiable data from the same company. But the overwhelming number of studies that were published as time wore on showed no benefit for patients taking hydroxychloroquine. In June 2020, the FDA abruptly revoked its approval and removed hydroxychloroquine from its emergency use status and revoked the emergency-use waiver that had been given to chloroquine as well. The agency took these actions because, according to its statement: "Based on FDA's continued review of the scientific evidence available for hydroxychloroquine sulfate (HCQ) and chloroquine phosphate (CQ) to treat COVID-19 ... FDA has determined that CQ and HCQ are unlikely to be effective in treating COVID-19."

Thus, current scientific evidence finds that hydroxy-chloroquine is not effective against COVID-19 and may pose a risk to heart function for some patients.

17. Is it safe to wear a mask? Will wearing one make me sick from breathing my own exhaled CO₂?

Masks are safe to wear, and they will not make an otherwise healthy person ill. Some people may find them restrictive, and people who suffer from anxiety may feel short of breath wearing one—but that's due to their anxiety, not the mask. Surgeons, nurses, and other health professionals routinely wear masks for hours at a time with no ill effects.

Social media memes have promoted the idea that masks won't protect you from the virus while simultaneously suggesting that they'll cause you to become ill from breathing your own exhaled carbon dioxide. These memes fail to take into account that molecules of carbon dioxide are considerably smaller than droplets that carry virus particles. A well-made mask can prevent the droplets from passing through the mask while still allowing air to flow through.

These memes have also fundamentally misunderstood *why* people should wear masks, however. "There is a common perception that wearing a facemask means you consider others a danger," said John Colvin, a researcher at the University of Greenwich, in a statement. "In fact, by wearing a mask, you are primarily protecting others from yourself. Cultural and even political issues may stop people from wearing facemasks, so the message needs to be clear: my mask protects you, your mask protects me." The goal isn't to keep others' respiratory droplets out of your mouth and nose (although a mask helps there too), it's to prevent *your* droplets from escaping to infect others, should you carry the virus. And given that COVID-19 doesn't always show itself in symptoms, you can't always know when you're infected—so a mask prevents you from infecting others during that phase where you're asymptomatic (see Question 17).

Scientists at the University of Cambridge and the University of Greenwich in the United Kingdom have demonstrated that widespread mask-wearing has a more potent reduction effect on coronavirus infection rates than widespread quarantines.

Indeed, population-wide use of face masks can force the **reproductive number** of a pandemic under 1.0, the researchers contend. The reproductive number, also known as **R0** (pronounced R-naught), is an epidemiological measure. It refers to the number of people to whom an infected individual can pass a virus. When the reproductive number is at 1.0, that means each infected person is passing the infection to one other person. R0 needs to stay under 1.0 for a pandemic to slow.

Reproductive number (R0)
The number of people to whom an infected individual can pass a virus.

In a series of modeling scenarios, the team of British researchers found that routine face mask use by 50% or more of a population can reduce viral transmission to an R value of less than 1.0. The study found that if people wear masks whenever they are in public, it is twice as effective at reducing the R value than if masks are worn only after symptoms appear.

Mask-wearing alone flattened future disease curves and additionally meant less stringent quarantine measures.

Despite these and other compelling studies, there was heated opposition to mask use in some parts of the United States. Dr. Nichole Quick, who had been the chief public health officer in Orange County, California, resigned her position during the pandemic after her recommendation for residents to wear face coverings in public sparked death threats and forced the local county government to provide a security detail for the doctor. Masks have become part of the culture wars that have divided the United States on a number of issues, including matters of public health.

18. Are the terms asymptomatic and presymptomatic just two sides of the same coin? It seems like they mean the same thing.

No, the two terms are fundamentally different—but before diving into an explanation, it should be noted that people in either of these categories can transmit their infection to others without having overt symptoms themselves.

Asymptomatic transmission

A communicable disease spread by someone who is harboring the virus but who will never develop the disease.

Asymptomatic carriers

People who are infected with a virus and capable of transmitting it to others but who do not develop disease symptoms.

Asymptomatic transmission means a communicable disease is spread by someone who is harboring the virus but who will never develop the signs or symptoms of the infectious disease, according to the CDC's definition of this group. These **asymptomatic carriers** can still make other people sick. Research on the prevalence of asymptomatic carriers, published in the *Annals of Internal Medicine*, suggests this group was likely of significant size in the early months of the COVID-19 pandemic, helping the contagion spread while not coming down with the disease themselves.

Authors of the report, Drs. Daniel P. Oran and Eric Topol of the Scripps Research Institute in California, estimated asymptomatic carriers to account for 40% to 45% of people infected with the virus. The report highlighted a need for expansive testing and contact tracing to mitigate transmission from this group of silent spreaders.

The concept of asymptomatic spread may seem confusing, but it has been documented in other kinds of communicable diseases. You may have heard of Mary Mallon, better known as "Typhoid Mary," who in the late 19th and early 20th centuries infected 47 people with the bacterium *Salmonella typhi*, which causes typhoid. Mallon worked as a cook for wealthy families in New York City and in the town of Oyster Bay on Long Island. Poor hand hygiene allowed her to pass the fecal bacteria to her employers and their families. There was no vaccine, and antibiotics had not yet been developed. Mallon's connection to the sickness was established and she was asked to isolate herself, but she angrily refused to, as it would prevent her from working; her continuing to work, however, meant more people got sick, and some of them died. As a result, the New York City Department of Health, which held enormous sway over its citizens in the early 1900s, arrested Mallon at gunpoint and banned her to North Brother Island in 1915. North Brother belongs to a tiny archipelago known at the time as the Quarantine Islands, off the city's coast. People with infectious diseases were sequestered for weeks, months—even decades—to prevent them from infecting others. Mallon remained there until her death in 1938. In total, she is believed to have infected at least 53 people with typhoid, but because she was uncooperative with investigators, the true number could be significantly higher. Typhoid Mary would be defined today as an asymptomatic carrier because the *Salmonella typhi* bacteria, which was confirmed by testing to be present in her body, never made her sick.

Presymptomatic transmission

Transmission of the virus during the time frame before infected individuals develop symptoms of illness.

Presymptomatic transmission, according to the CDC, refers to individuals who transmit coronavirus infections when they are not exhibiting symptoms, but later go on to develop COVID-19. Presymptomatic individuals are not mere carriers—they're people who are infected and will eventually become sick, but who haven't yet started to display symptoms (it's worth pointing out that presymptomatic periods for COVID-19 have been documented to be as long as two weeks, which is a considerable time for people to walk around thinking they're healthy and interacting with others according to that belief). Transmission can occur between people who are in close proximity, engaging in conversation, or singing in a choir. Coughs and sneezes, of course, are more powerful, producing more droplet sprays that travel farther. Social distancing recommendations are predicated on 6 feet of separation to avoid being infected with viral particles expelled in aerosols and sprays. As discussed in Question 11, some scientists have discovered that coughs and sneezes launch droplets farther than the 6-foot rule.

19. Are men more likely to have poor outcomes than women with COVID-19?

Studies suggest that, yes, men do indeed have worse outcomes than women. Medical analyses in the United States and elsewhere have documented higher morbidity and mortality among men diagnosed with COVID-19. For example, a study published in the April 22, 2020, edition of the *Journal of the American Medical Association*

(*JAMA*) revealed striking differences among people who survived or died after a COVID-19 diagnosis.

The research, which involved 5,700 men and women treated for coronavirus infections in New York City, found that male mortality exceeded that of women in all age categories. The greater New York City metropolitan area was the initial epicenter of U.S. COVID-19 infections. The findings apparently were not a fluke, because stark gender disparities have been reported in a flurry of COVID-19 studies from throughout the world. Older people in general are more likely to succumb to the disease, but older men, particularly those in their 80s, are more likely to succumb to the disease than older women.

Men with comorbidities were also more than twice as likely to die of COVID-19 as women.

In Italy, doctors who also reported their findings in *JAMA* zeroed in on yet another difference: 82% of 1,591 admissions to intensive care units (ICUs) were men. The analysis focused on patients treated in Lombardy, which was hard hit by COVID-19. The ICU admissions suggested that patients who suffered severe complications were more likely to be men than women. But these discoveries should come as no surprise, because male vulnerability had been documented years earlier in patients infected with the other two coronavirus diseases, SARS and MERS.

As disheartening as the data may seem, the reports are probably not the final word. Men diagnosed with coronavirus disease are not necessarily destined to die. Many survive—and thrive—after diagnosis. Some men who test positive develop no symptoms at all. But while no study is predictive of what happens in every case, the research does provide clarity for doctors and patients on gender disparities.

That said, some scientists have suggested the difference in coronavirus outcomes centers on maleness itself. Medical investigators at Albert Einstein College of Medicine in the Bronx, New York, suggest SARS-CoV-2 (the virus that causes COVID-19) collects in the testicles, which become a reservoir of viral persistence. The study was posted on the medRxiv site, which allows researchers to publish their work without the benefit of peer review. It is possible that the study, which was a collaborative one with another team in India, may one day be published in a major medical journal.

Not having one's research published in a peer-reviewed scientific journal doesn't mean the research is without merit. The analysis bases its reasoning on a compelling fact: The testes are among sites in the human body where cells are studded with ACE2 receptors, the protein that the virus uses to enter cells and infect them.

As it turns out, there is a previous link to SARS and the testes. In a 2006 study reported in the journal *Biology of Reproduction*, scientists in China found that SARS caused orchitis, a condition in which the testicles become inflamed.

20. Didn't hot weather kill SARS? So shouldn't warm weather also destroy the virus that causes COVID-19?

No, hot weather didn't kill SARS. That myth is one of the most enduring fallacies that has lingered since the deadly SARS episode ended in the early 2000s. The idea that warm temperatures would stop the COVID-19 pandemic was revived as coronavirus infections began to circumnavigate the globe.

Because so many people believed that warm weather destroyed SARS, they hoped the same would come true for COVID-19. These notions were stoked by President Trump in March 2020, when he told a group of governors: "A lot of people think that this goes away in April with the heat. As the heat comes in, typically [the coronavirus] will go away in April."

His words came as the virus had already made its way to the African continent—Egypt's first case occurred in February. In time, no country in the Southern Hemisphere where temperatures are warm year-round would be left untouched by COVID-19. Countries below the equator were as vulnerable to the pandemic virus as nations in the Northern Hemisphere. Brazil became a major South American epicenter of the infection; its gravediggers can barely keep up with the mounting pace of COVID-19 deaths.

Still, the myth about SARS and warm weather persisted despite evidence to the contrary. "SARS did not die of natural causes," wrote Dr. Marc Lipsitch in an article on the website of the Center for Communicable Disease Dynamics at Harvard's T.H. Chan School of Public Health. "It was killed by extremely intense public health interventions in mainland Chinese cities, Hong Kong, Vietnam, Thailand, Canada, and elsewhere." Lipsitch is the Center's director, and he emphasized that very stringent measures were what drove SARS out of circulation: "These involved isolating cases, quarantining their contacts, a measure of 'social distancing,' and other intensive efforts. These worked well for SARS because those who were most infectious were also quite ill in a distinctive way—the sick cases were the transmitters, so isolating the sick curbed transmission."

It was not easy to snuff out an infectious disease from a virus that was circulating in humans for the first time. "In Toronto, SARS resurged after the initial wave was controlled and precautions were discontinued," Lipsitch recalled. "This resurgence was linked to a case from the first wave. The resurgence confirms that it was control measures that stopped transmission the first time."

PART THREE

Understanding Outbreaks, Epidemics, and Pandemics

What is the difference between an outbreak, an epidemic, and a pandemic?

Does the word epidemic refer only to infectious diseases?

What do epidemiologists mean when they say we need to "flatten the curve"?

More . . .

21. What is the difference between an outbreak, an epidemic, and a pandemic?

Outbreak

A greater-than-expected increase of a disease in a population.

Epidemic

A disease that affects a large number of people in a community; in the case of an infectious disease, sustained transmission is an epidemic hallmark.

In strict epidemiological terms, an **outbreak** refers to a a greater-than-expected increase of a disease in a population, but in a more limited geographic area than an epidemic. An **epidemic** is a sudden and rapid increase of a disease that affects a large number of people in a population, and in the case of an infectious disease, like COVID-19, sustained disease transmission is an epidemic hallmark. The population in an epidemic may involve a large number of people in a town, or county. An epidemic may even affect a state or group of states, or an entire country. An epidemic becomes a pandemic when the disease spreads to multiple countries and continents. Another way to look at it: A pandemic is an epidemic that travels.

The respiratory illnesses that emerged suddenly in Wuhan, China, in the winter of 2019 started as a local outbreak. In December, when the late Dr. Li Wenliang, the Wuhan ophthalmologist who first reported the outbreak, sounded his alarm to colleagues about SARS-like respiratory infections, he reported only seven cases. But community spread of the disease was already underway and would soon explode into a full-blown epidemic. Experts in infectious diseases in the United States and elsewhere in the world who were observing China from afar correctly guessed that a novel virus was probably the cause. A new pathogen is a jolting thought because it invariably suggests that a pandemic could likely unfold.

22. Does the word epidemic refer only to infectious diseases?

There was a time when the term *epidemic* was a word that primarily defined infectious diseases because communicable conditions were widespread; epidemics were common and frequently deadly. In the 19th century, yellow fever epidemics plagued many regions of the United States. Polio epidemics were a feared seasonal menace throughout the first half of the 20th century until vaccines came along in the 1950s and forever erased a once expected summertime contagion. The list goes on: Scarlet fever, measles, and chickenpox were other noteworthy infectious causes of epidemics, and perhaps a reason the word epidemic was tightly bound to infectious diseases. Even now, flu epidemics occur somewhere in the world every year.

But the word epidemic has taken on broader meaning over the years to include conditions that are not contagious. You very likely have heard of the opioid epidemic, the obesity epidemic, the suicide epidemic, and the homelessness epidemic. Epidemiologists who study these conditions ask many of the same questions that are asked in studies of infectious diseases: What size is the affected population, and how fast is the epidemic growing?

23. What do epidemiologists mean when they say we need to "flatten the curve"?

Terminology that was once arcane and limited to the research of biostatisticians has made its way into daily usage as a result of the coronavirus pandemic. **Flattening the epidemic curve** is one of those terms. It means stopping new infections from developing, hence reducing the overall number of cases. When infections are reduced, not only are lives saved, but a huge burden is lifted off hospitals, which operate more efficiently—and not

Flattening the epidemic curve

A biostatistics term that means stopping new infections from developing and thereby reducing the overall number of cases.

beyond capacity—when there are fewer cases to treat. Imagine the curve as a bell. Flattening it simply means reducing cases to make the bell-shaped curve less steep.

New York's Governor Andrew Cuomo frequently used the term in daily news briefings during the height of the COVID-19 crisis in his state. New York was the U.S. epicenter of the disease for weeks. Over a period of several weeks, as many as 700 to 800 people were dying daily in New York City alone. Although some residents vehemently opposed the restrictions of "sheltering in place," which meant staying at home, New York's State Department of Health found that the effort helped drive down the COVID-19 infection rate. The benefit came from simple nonpharmaceutical measures, such as not going to work or school, and avoiding theaters, sports arenas, and other entertainment venues. Church services became virtual gatherings in cyberspace, as were meetings for most businesses.

Social distancing

The practice of staying at least 6 feet away from other people to reduce the potential for virus transmission.

To flatten a curve, each individual must literally stay out of the path of the virus. **Social distancing**—staying 6 feet away from others in public—frequent handwashing and wearing a mask in public proved to be effective strategies in a pandemic.

Herd immunity

Also called community immunity, which occurs when enough people in a community are immune to an infectious disease making its spread unlikely. Herd immunity is achieved through vaccination.

24. What is "herd immunity"? Could herd immunity have prevented COVID-19 from spreading?

Herd immunity occurs when a large percentage of a population is immune to an infectious disease. The infectious agent can't gain a foothold in the population because too many people can thwart it. In *Gordis Epidemiology*, a leading textbook, the authors write: "Once a certain proportion of people in the community are immune, the likelihood is small that an infected person will encounter a susceptible person to whom the infection can be transmitted." In such a situation, vulnerable individuals are, in effect, protected by the immunity of those around them (the "herd" in herd immunity). Vaccination is the primary intervention that helps create herd immunity. In the era before the measles vaccine existed, it was well known that each person who developed the viral infection was capable of spreading it to at least 10 to 15 other people. With that kind of transmission potential, a few cases could quickly ignite an epidemic. To achieve herd immunity among school-aged children for measles, public health officials now know that 90% to 95% of this population needs to be vaccinated against the infection. For less contagious communicable diseases, the vaccination rate doesn't have to be quite as high. To achieve herd immunity for polio, the vaccination rate needs to be in the 80% to 85% range. Herd immunity is important in public health because it means an entire population doesn't have to be vaccinated for a community to achieve herd immunity. This is especially important for people in the population who are immune-deficient because they are newborns or of advanced age; have cancer, or other immune-compromising conditions.

Unfortunately, in order to develop herd immunity without the benefit of a vaccine, an enormous number of people first have to become infected with the virus so they can develop immunity. When a virus has the lethal potential of SARS-CoV-2, this is a risky strategy; it means putting people who may have hidden vulnerabilities into harm's way. Anders Tegnell, the physician who created Sweden's COVID-19 strategy, felt that this was a risk worth taking. Based on Tegnell's plan, Sweden kept its schools and businesses open and gatherings of up to 50 people were allowed. His theory was anchored in the notion that the hale and hearty would contract the infection, recover, and become immune to the infection, providing a safety net that would protect the vulnerable.

The trouble with Tegnell's strategy is that it didn't work out as planned. Sweden wound up with infection and death rates that were higher than its Scandinavian neighbors. By early June, Tegnell told Swedish Radio that in hindsight, it may not have been the best plan. "If we were to run into the same disease knowing exactly what we know about it today, I think we would end up doing something in between what Sweden did and what the rest of the world has done," he commented.

25. What is a Public Health Emergency of International Concern?

Public Health Emergency of International Concern (PHEIC)

A formal declaration by the WHO to highlight an extraordinary public health event that poses a risk to other countries.

A **Public Health Emergency of International Concern** or PHEIC is a formal declaration by the WHO to highlight an extraordinary public health event—such as a growing infectious disease outbreak—that poses a risk to other countries. The declaration is not made by an individual but is determined by a panel of outside experts that WHO convenes. Panelists assess the threat and determine by a majority vote whether the declaration should be made.

In 2019, a PHEIC was declared because of the Ebola epidemic in the Democratic Republic of the Congo. Ongoing disease transmission in that country posed an international threat, panelists concluded with their votes. The declaration conveys power to the WHO

Director-General to advise other countries about border closures, air travel, and the need for a coordinated international response. A PHEIC was declared in the COVID-19 outbreak on January 30, 2020, roughly a month after Dr. Li Wenliang, a Wuhan doctor (see Question 32), warned other physicians that patients were quarantined at the hospital where he worked. All had been diagnosed with an atypical pneumonia that resembled SARS. Dr. Tedros Adhanom Ghebreyesus, WHO's Director-General, announced the PHEIC at a news conference. "This declaration is not a vote of no confidence in China," Tedros said, noting that the emergency meant it was time for international solidarity.

26. Does the World Health Organization determine when an epidemic becomes a pandemic?

Just as the WHO declares a PHEIC, it also determines when an epidemic becomes a global pandemic. COVID-19 was declared a pandemic on March 11, 2020. By that time, it had spread to more than 100 countries. As he announced the declaration, Dr. Tedros, Director-General of the WHO, warned countries that the situation would worsen.

On the day the pandemic was declared, there were 118,000 confirmed cases worldwide and 4,300 deaths had been counted. Tedros was criticized on social media for having waited until March to officially declare a pandemic. Critics said the determination should have been made weeks earlier. The embattled Director-General was also lambasted by detractors who claimed he was coddling China, which was accused of downplaying the seriousness of its epidemic.

Tedros, who is Ethiopian, is the first black Director-General of the World Health Organization. He received a steady stream of death threats and racist comments during the early weeks of the pandemic. He addressed the attacks during a WHO news briefing about a month after the pandemic was officially declared. "I can tell you, personal attacks have been going on for more than two, three months," Tedros said, describing the slurs and threats. He concluded his remarks by saying: "I don't give a damn," referring to what his detractors said about him. Tedros said his main focus was the pandemic.

U.S. President Donald Trump was one of the Director-General's staunchest critics. In April, Trump said he was pulling U.S. funding out of the World Health Organization. It was estimated that the United States contributed more than $400 million annually to the global health organization. Trump's decision was rebuked by his critics as an effort to deflect attention from the weak federal response as the pandemic spread in the United States (see Question 28). By the spring of 2020, the U.S. had become the country with the largest number of confirmed cases and highest number of deaths globally.

27. What were the major pandemics of the 20th century?

There were three major, globe-circling pandemics that killed millions of people in the last century. Each stands out in global health history providing valuable lessons for epidemiologists who are studying pandemics today, especially the COVID-19 pandemic.

1. The pandemic influenza of 1918—sometimes called the Spanish flu, or as the title of author

John Barry's 2004 book described it, *The Great Influenza*—occurred in three waves, which were plotted on graphs at the time. (Even though people to this day refer to the 1918 pandemic as the Spanish flu, it didn't begin in Spain. The term has been misleading historians for more than a century.) The 1918 flu pandemic was spawned by an H1N1 flu virus, identified decades after the pandemic. It killed more people than World War I did. Virologists today say this H1N1 strain was uniquely lethal. A conservative estimate suggests that 50 million people died worldwide, but the death toll may have been as high as 100 million, because the flu spread throughout countries that lacked modern methods of disease surveillance. The United States, European nations, China, Japan, and Australia had relatively accurate data on the number of people who succumbed, but the story was different elsewhere in the world. Native Americans who lived in remote Arctic villages were decimated by the flu. An estimated 17 million people died in India. The infection infiltrated Ethiopia's royal court, infecting Haile Selassie, who survived the flu and later became emperor. Medical scientists in 1918 had no idea what kind of pathogen caused the devastating waves of illness, even though they were well aware of the extreme contagiousness. In the United States, public health officials ordered an array of interventions to prevent the spread of influenza, such as requiring people to wear masks, closing schools and businesses, and halting church services. Some communities were better at implementing these measures than others and as a result were able to spare more lives.

2. In 1957, the pandemic flu strain H2N2 emerged and was named the Asian flu because its origins were traced to Asia. An estimated two million people died worldwide. Global health authorities suspected a pandemic was developing when 250,000 cases of influenza quickly swept through Hong Kong. Scientists in the United States and the United Kingdom collaborated in a major scientific effort to isolate and identify the virus. Team members discovered they were witnessing a virus that had undergone antigenic shift. This means they had identified a flu virus whose surface proteins, hemagglutinin (HA) and neuraminidase (NA), were unlike any other in circulation. Flu viruses that emerge as a result of **antigenic shift** can result in a novel influenza A subtype that has never before challenged the human immune system. The discovery was a signal to the international collaborators that they were dealing with a pandemic strain.

3. The 1968 Hong Kong flu is another pandemic with a name that does not quite reflect its origin. This flu virus is believed to have originated in Southeast Asia and was caused by an H3N2 flu virus. An estimated one million people died worldwide. Descendants of this virus now circulate as seasonal flu.

Antigenic shift

A change in the surface proteins of a virus that renders it unfamiliar to the human immune system, making it highly infectious, with potential to become a pandemic virus.

28. How have U.S. presidents responded to pandemics?

President Joe Biden was faced with an explosive public health disaster and nationwide economic decline by the time he assumed office in January 2021. His transition to power arrived just two weeks after a deadly insurrection raged on Capitol Hill, led by a mob of angry Trump supporters attempting to overturn the results of the 2020 election. Five people died. Biden proposed a $1.9 trillion COVID relief and economic stimulus package, which had multiple aims. The thrust of his plan was to steer the United States out of the pandemic after a year of gross mismanagement of the crisis under the Trump administration. The United States, the richest nation in the world, outpaced the entire planet in the number coronavirus cases and deaths. By the time Biden assumed office, new variants of the virus had also begun spreading in multiple states, including California where a unique U.S. variant, CAL.20C, another spike protein mutation, had emerged.

The Biden plan's centerpiece was the use of the Defense Production Act to ramp up vaccine production with an aim of 100 million vaccinations across the United States in 100 days. The Act became law during the Korean War era and gives the nation's chief executive broad powers over U.S. businesses. The Act authorizes the president to prioritize the production of materials deemed vital to national defense. In the case of the pandemic, President Biden prioritized the production of vaccines and all required accessory equipment (vials and syringes) to accomplish the sweeping inoculation plan.

He also called for a nationwide corps of "vaccinators," people who could administer the shots, such as retired doctors and nurses as well as specially trained military personnel. The president also put an emphasis on science in his administration by rejoining the World Health Organization and creating the role of Presidential Science Advisor as a new cabinet-level position. Dr. Eric Lander, director of the Broad Institute, a joint research effort between Harvard University and MIT, was named to the post.

President Trump declared a public health emergency in January 2020 under the Public Health Service Act and issued two national emergency declarations under the Stafford Act and the National Emergencies Act, but beyond that, his administration did little to support states battling the pandemic as it spread, with New York City being hit very hard, as discussed in Question 23. The president took the position that individual states needed to take the lead in containing the virus, which led to an unfortunate lack of nationwide coordination—some states, such as Maine and Hawaii, quickly initiated stringent lockdown approaches, while others, such as Florida and Arizona, did not. States also found themselves competing for essential supplies with other states and sometimes with the federal government itself. In the midst of it all, the Trump Administration dramatically diminished the functions of the CDC and eliminated its role as the central, coordinating agency for major disease outbreaks. The CDC's decades-long preparation for a global pandemic was lost as the largest pandemic in 102 years unfolded.

This response stands in marked contrast to how previous presidents handled pandemics and epidemics. In 2009, President Barack Obama declared H1N1 flu a public health emergency 6 weeks before it was officially defined as a pandemic. Six months later, he declared a national emergency. The CDC, in its summary of the U.S. 2009 pandemic strategy, described it as complex, multifaceted, and long term. The CDC was also mobilized five years later in response to the Ebola epidemic in West Africa, even though its impact on the United States was minimal. The Obama administration additionally established the National Security Council Directorate for Global Health Security and Biodefense, a special White House team whose role was to monitor and provide guidance on infectious disease threats. The directorate was dissolved by the Trump administration in 2018.

Under President George W. Bush, the CDC activated its emergency operation center on March 14, 2003, shortly after SARS was identified. The agency also issued a series of travel alerts, cautioning Americans about affected countries. On March 28, the CDC implemented its national pandemic plan for SARS.

In 1968, President Lyndon Johnson was too sick with the Hong Kong flu to have played much of a role in national planning. He commented that it was one of the worst illnesses that he had ever experienced. Nevertheless, the CDC—then called the National Communicable Disease Center—played a role in coordinating state public health officials who were monitoring the spread of the illness.

President Dwight Eisenhower in 1957 refused to call for a national vaccination strategy, even as the Asian flu spread across the country. Historians say Eisenhower felt that vaccination plans should be left to private enterprises. However, the head of respiratory diseases at Walter Reed Army Institute of Research, Maurice Hilleman, recognized the danger and coordinated an effort to develop a vaccine so quickly that by the time the Asian flu began to spread in the United States, a vaccine was ready.

It's interesting to note that another president, Woodrow Wilson, took a similar approach to President Trump's when confronted with the 1918 pandemic. Wilson disregarded information from his medical advisers during the 1918 pandemic and sent troops to war despite expanding outbreaks in parts of the United States and abroad. Like President Trump, he left the pandemic response mostly to local authorities, so that the impact varied widely from one community to the next. As mentioned in Question 27, the differences in approach have been highlighted in the form of graphs comparing the successful response by the city of St. Louis, involving early and aggressive shutdowns and quarantines, versus the slower, less aggressive, and ultimately less successful response by Philadelphia.

29. Did the 1918 pandemic occur in waves? If so, how many waves were there?

Most contemporary epidemiologists estimate that a series of waves characterized the 1918 global flu pandemic. The first wave occurred in the spring of 1918, the second in the fall of that year, then in some countries—but not all—a third wave ignited illnesses in the early part of 1919. The initial spring wave arose at a time of year that is not favorable to influenza's spread. The calamitous second wave, however, caused simultaneous outbreaks in the Northern and Southern Hemispheres, sweeping violently through populations from September to November. An equally violent third wave continued through the early months of 1919. By the end of spring in 1919, the pandemic had run its course.

30. Do individual U.S. states have pandemic plans?

Most states crafted pandemic plans in the early 2000s. The primary aim was to prepare for a flu pandemic. Yet, when COVID-19 began sickening people across the country, the responses differed from state to state. Some states seemed to have no formal response to the pandemic at all. Worse, there was no central coordination.

The U.S. Centers for Disease Control and Prevention, which had been weakened under the Trump administration, was not in a position to oversee and advise states, which has been its traditional role for decades. The CDC did not hold daily news briefings in 2020, sessions that would have allowed for reports on surveillance, hospital capacity statistics, case counts, deaths, and other vital information.

31. Is it true that epidemics are inevitable, but pandemics are avoidable?

As unimaginable as it may seem, the answer is yes. Infectious disease epidemics occur frequently, especially those caused by influenza viruses, which circulate seasonally. It is uncertain as of this writing whether COVID-19 will become seasonal.

Pandemics used to be considered relatively rare events. As noted earlier in this chapter, only three occurred in the last century. But with three early in this century—two caused by novel coronaviruses and one by a novel A strain of flu—it's time for the world to take pandemics seriously. It is also time to consider **pandemic forecasting**.

Some scientists suggest that international governments should collaborate on forming a global surveillance system. The aim would be to predict pandemics the way the National Oceanic and Atmospheric Administration

Pandemic forecasting

A proposed system of surveillance to identify infectious diseases with pandemic potential when they first emerge, with the goal of preventing pandemics.

(NOAA) accurately forecasts hurricanes. Knowing where the hotspots are would allow mitigation efforts to be organized. Outbreaks could be extinguished before they erupt out of control. Dr. Michael Lu, dean of the School of Public Health at the University of California at Berkeley, spelled out that possibility in an essay published in *The Washington Post*. He suggests that accurate forecasting is needed to spare lives and economies.

Another possibility is to get a better handle on some of the zoonotic viruses still lurking in the environment. That's a tall order. More than 800,000 viruses are believed to be harbored by animals in the wild—and these pathogens have yet to be discovered. Dr. Peter Daszak, president of EcoHealth Alliance, is a virus hunter whose job it is to do just that: find viruses before they find us. Daszak published the first global emerging disease hotspot map, and in collaboration with scientists in China, identified the bat origin of SARS.

But virus hunting is not universally appreciated, especially in a world with a growing population of science deniers who don't appreciate the value of objective scientific facts. Daszak was part of a team that was isolating previously unknown bat coronaviruses and sequencing their genes when the Trump administration abruptly cut the team's funding in 2020.

32. If China's government had not forced the Wuhan whistleblower to claim that COVID-19 was a rumor, could a pandemic have been avoided?

It is difficult to say what would have happened in China if authorities had taken a less aggressive stance toward

Dr. Li Wenliang. But given that he sounded his alarm on December 31, it's unlikely that his message about a SARS-like disease would have averted Wuhan's outbreak or the global pandemic that would soon ensue.

Li, who died of COVID-19 in February 2020, was an ophthalmologist at Wuhan Central Hospital. He is credited as the first person to alert other doctors about an unusual pneumonia in local Wuhan patients. The disease, he told them, was frighteningly reminiscent of SARS. Li didn't send his post to a large number of people. He messaged members of his medical school alumni group on WeChat, a social media platform, saying seven people from a local seafood market had symptoms of SARS-like pneumonia. All were quarantined at Wuhan Central Hospital. In a late January interview with *The New York Times* from his hospital bed, Li wrote via WeChat that he knew the disease was dangerous when one of his patients infected her entire family and him as well.

For him, trouble with authorities started in early January when the message sent to alumni members was reposted by someone. It spread like wildfire. Unfortunately, his name was still visible, and police caught wind of it. They commanded him to come to a local Wuhan station, where Li was reprimanded for spreading rumors.

The doctor was forced to sign a document acknowledging that he had distributed a rumor. The public understanding of the situation as a result of that document was that they had nothing to worry about. All of this began to unravel as 2020 dawned. COVID-19 was already spreading; Li himself would be dead of the disease in a matter of weeks. His plight nevertheless captured the hearts and minds of many. He was hailed as a hero, and upon his death the country unofficially went into national mourning. China Global Television Network (CGTN) broadcast dozens of stories about the young doctor and always referred to him as the whistleblower.

PART FOUR

Children and Coronaviruses

How vulnerable are children to COVID-19?

What are the symptoms of COVID-19 in children?

What are some of the complications of
COVID-19 in children?

More . . .

33. How vulnerable are children to COVID-19?

Few pandemic concerns about COVID-19 have engendered more discussion—and misinformation—than the issue of pediatric susceptibility to COVID-19. Claims by politicians that children are immune to infection are patently false. Children have a lower risk than adults, but their risk isn't zero.

Epidemiological data

Data related to how and in whom a disease spreads.

Here are the facts: **Epidemiological data** from the Centers for Disease Control and Prevention (CDC) confirm there have been fewer cases of COVID-19 among children age 0 to 17, compared with people who are older than 18, suggesting that COVID-19 is largely a disease of adults—but not exclusively so. For example, statistics compiled by the CDC show that 7.3% of more than 5 million confirmed COVID-19 cases in the United States occurred among children under age 18 in the first 8 months of the pandemic. Kids in this age group make up 22% of the total U.S. population. The American Academy of Pediatrics and the Children's Hospital Association, nevertheless, found in their research that children represent about 9% of all COVID-19 cases in the United States.

Disease burden

An estimate of the proportion of a population that is affected by a disease.

Regardless of how the statistics are parsed, there is a comparatively lower percentage of pediatric cases in the United States, and that correlates with what other countries have also found: a lower COVID-19 **disease burden** among children. Few pediatric cases were documented in studies examining outbreaks of SARS and MERS, two other serious infections caused by coronaviruses. To get a better understanding of the SARS era, during which adults died at an alarmingly high rate, a 2007 Canadian analysis published in *The Pediatric*

Infectious Disease Journal, reported that children with SARS, 12 years of age or younger, had only mild disease. Younger children were less likely than older kids to be admitted to hospital intensive care, receive supplemental oxygen, or be treated with methylprednisolone, a steroid drug to reduce inflammation. During the fleeting SARS era, which ran from the fall of 2002 to the summer of 2003, there was no disease manifestation comparable to multisystem inflammatory syndrome in children (MIS-C), a rare but severe inflammatory condition in youngsters that emerged during the first few months of the COVID-19 pandemic. Some doctors theorize that the lower pediatric infection rate and milder course of infection may have been a result of exposure to coronaviruses that cause the common cold.

The vast majority of pediatric COVID-19 cases are believed to be mild or **asymptomatic**, but there remain countless unknowns about the infection when it comes to kids. Although CDC epidemiologists detected a steady rise in childhood infections with SARS-CoV-2 from spring through summer of 2020, they underscored that the true **incidence** of infection during the early months of the pandemic remains unknown due to a variety of factors. Chief among them is a lack of pediatric data from **antibody testing**. Insufficient screenings were conducted among children, the CDC has stated, noting the vast majority of testing programs throughout the United States focused on adults.

That said, medical scientists are convinced that most cases among children don't cause serious symptoms because substantially lower rates of pediatric hospitalization suggest this pivotal population is capable of harboring and spreading the virus while, for the most part, escaping its most devastating consequences.

Asymptomatic
Lack of disease symptoms in a person who nonetheless is infected.

Incidence
The number of new cases of a disease within a specific population during a set time period.

Antibody testing
Tests that identify whether antibodies specific to a particular infectious agent are present in a person's blood.

CDC and WHO data suggest children probably carry the same or higher nasopharyngeal **viral load**—the amount of virus in their nasal passages and throats—as adults. Both agencies also agree that the **incubation period** for children is essentially the same as it is for adults: 2 to 14 days with an average of about 6 days.

While some medical experts have questioned whether children transmit the virus as effectively as adults, other clinicians have pointed to outbreaks and clusters of SARS-CoV-2 in summer camps and schools. Anecdotal evidence abounds of American summer camps and K–12 schools in Europe, Israel, and South Africa having to close because children—and teaching staff—tested positive for the virus. The CDC's COVID-19-NET Surveillance team, which has studied epidemiology of COVID-19 in children, has urged the reinforcement of prevention efforts—hand-washing, physical distancing, and masks—in **congregate settings** that serve children, including childcare centers, camps, and schools. Failing to adhere to hygiene measures can escalate infection risks at home should children expose family members to an infection picked up at school. A similar school-to-home infection pipeline has been documented for years in the spread of influenza.

Pulitzer Prize-winning science journalist Laurie Garrett, writing in *Foreign Policy*, emphasized that pediatric SARS-CoV-2 asymptomatic carriers can put at risk their parents and grandparents—populations more likely to suffer serious bouts of the infection. "A South Korean government survey of 60,000 households discovered that adults living in households that had an infected child aged 10 to 19 years had the highest rate of catching the coronavirus," Garrett reported. "Nearly 19 percent of people living with an infected teenager went

Viral load

The amount of virus in the body.

Incubation period

The time from initial exposure to an infectious disease to the appearance of symptoms that indicate a person has been infected.

Congregate settings

Places or situations where people gather together in large groups, such as schools, summer camps, or places of worship.

on to test positive for the virus within 10 days." She additionally referenced a nonprofit group's research, which highlighted risks for multigenerational households. "A Kaiser Family Foundation study says some 3.3 million adults over 65 in the United States live in a home with at least one school-aged child," Garrett wrote, underscoring that grandparents are put at risk when precautions are not heeded in schools.

An analysis of pediatric COVID-19 cases from March to July 2020 in 14 hospitals across the United States emphasized the importance of tracking pediatric SARS-CoV-2 infections to highlight how children are affected. A small but worrisome percentage of children are hospitalized, and a fraction of those children are admitted to intensive care units. The infection also can be fatal for some children. Writing in the CDC's *Morbidity and Mortality Weekly Report*, members of the CDC's COVID-19-Associated Hospitalization Surveillance Network (COVID-NET Surveillance team) say that even though exposure often means an asymptomatic case for most children, "less is known about severe COVID-19 in children requiring hospitalization."

34. What are the symptoms of COVID-19 in children?

The **signs and symptoms** of COVID-19 in children are similar to those in adults. Some parents have said they initially thought their child was coming down with a cold. The CDC lists the following symptoms:

- Fever
- Fatigue
- Headache
- Muscle pain

Signs and symptoms

Indicators of the presence of disease. Signs are measurable, observable indicators (fever, rash), while symptoms are subjective (fatigue, pain).

- Cough
- Nasal congestion
- New loss of taste or smell
- Sore throat
- Shortness of breath or difficulty breathing
- Abdominal pain
- Diarrhea
- Nausea or vomiting
- Poor appetite or poor feeding

Doctors say the most common symptoms among children are cough and/or fever.

35. Are children hospitalized for COVID-19?

As mentioned in Question 33, most children who become infected with SARS-CoV-2 develop a mild case or are asymptomatic, but some kids develop infections that are serious enough to warrant hospitalization. The 14-state pediatric research project conducted by the COVID-NET group at the CDC found the rate of hospitalization among children under the age of 18 to be 8.0 per every 100,000 people in the population. That compares with 164.5 per 100,000 for adults. The data covered hospitalizations from March 1 to July 25, 2020, involving 576 children whose median age was 8. The gender divide was almost even, with boys representing 50.7% of the study cohort. By age group, children between 12 and 17 made up the study's largest number of COVID-19 patients, accounting for 241 of the 576 kids (41%) confined to hospitals. The second-largest group was the youngest and most vulnerable: babies, age 0 to 2 months, who made up 18.8% of hospitalized patients, or 108 of the 576.

One of the standout findings involved the sickest children. Among youngsters hospitalized for COVID-19, 1 in 3 had to be admitted to an **intensive care unit (ICU)** for treatment of complications. Pediatric ICU admissions, the researchers found, were comparable to those for adults. An estimated 1 in 3 adults hospitalized for COVID-19 have been admitted to an ICU.

A significant number of the hospitalized children—42%—had co-morbidities. The most prevalent conditions included obesity, which affected 38.7% of the children, chronic lung conditions, such as asthma, affected 18%, and prematurity (a gestational age of less than 37 weeks) affected 15.4%.

Among children who had a chest X-ray during hospitalization, 65.7% had what doctors referred to as **consolidation**, which means fluid in lung spaces that should be filled with air. For those who received CT scans, doctors reported obvious evidence of infection. Investigational treatments were administered to only 12 of the children; nine were infused with the antiviral drug **remdesivir**. Clinical trial data have shown that remdesivir can expedite recovery.

Even though pediatric hospitalizations involved children of all ethnicities, Latino and Black children were hospitalized at a higher rate than white children under the age of 18. The COVID-NET research analysis found that 16.4 Latino children per 100,000 people in the population were hospitalized for COVID-19; Black children were hospitalized at a rate of 10.5 per 100,000. The rate of hospitalization for Latino children was nearly eight times the rate of hospitalization for white children. For Black pediatric patients, the hospitalization rate was five times that of white children.

Intensive care unit (ICU)
A hospital department that gives continual monitoring and high-level care to extremely sick patients.

Consolidation
Fluid in lung spaces that should be filled with air.

Remdesivir
An antiviral drug, originally developed as a potential treatment for hepatitis C, but used in a number of viral infections. It has been given an emergency authorization by the FDA for use in COVID-19 treatment. The WHO cautions that patients hospitalized with COVID-19 should not be given remdesivir.

"Reasons for disparities in COVID-19-associated hospitalization rates by race and ethnicity are not fully understood," the COVID-NET team wrote in the discussion portion of their research analysis. The research team suggested one possibility: a greater prevalence of parents who work in essential occupations, a factor that might explain the higher incidence of COVID-19 among minority group children. A parent's exposure to the virus at work could likely mean **secondary transmission** to family members at home. During the 2009 flu pandemic, which wasn't nearly as pervasive as the global COVID-19 pandemic, a similar pattern of higher morbidity was reported among ethnic minority children.

Secondary transmission

The transmission of the virus to others by an index patient, who may (or may not be) asymptomatic.

36. Are babies affected by COVID-19?

In the study by the CDC's COVID-NET team, 188 of the hospitalized patients were babies 23 months and younger; the majority (108) of the patients were age 0 to 2 months. Although infant infections are rare, an emerging body of research suggests that babies who become infected are at elevated risk of serious illness with COVID-19.

Newborns and even somewhat older babies have immature immune systems and have not developed resilience against common afflictions, let alone a new pandemic disease. By contrast, older children have more robust immune systems, which have been tested and bolstered through bouts with the common cold, the flu, and a variety of microbial disease exposures that occur in the normal whirlwind of life.

Newborns can become infected in a variety of ways: during childbirth or when being handled by an infected mother or clinician at a hospital. At home, infected visitors or older siblings may transmit the infection. A case study in *The Pediatric Infectious Disease Journal* suggests SARS-CoV-2 can reach young lives in yet another way—by crossing the placenta during gestation.

Medical investigators at the University of Texas Southwestern Medical Center who reported the case study described a newborn as having tested positive for SARS-CoV-2. The mother's infection with the virus was confirmed by way of a nasal swab test. SARS-CoV-2 is not associated with brain impairment or neurological problems that are associated with other viruses that cross the placenta, such as Zika and rubella.

New mothers who have tested positive for the coronavirus are advised to wear a mask and to be fastidious about hand hygiene. There is no evidence, meanwhile, that the virus is transmitted through breast milk. Scientists at the University of California, San Diego, examined 64 samples of breast milk collected from the Mommy's Milk: Human Milk Research Biorepository. The samples had been collected from 18 women across the United States; all were infected with SARS-CoV-2. One sample tested positive for viral RNA, which is not infectious. Additional tests revealed there were no replicating viruses in the sample. Scientists concluded that breast milk is an unlikely mode of SARS-CoV-2 transmission.

37. What are some of the complications of COVID-19 in children?

Although **pre-existing conditions** have complicated COVID-19 for children who were hospitalized, as mentioned in Question 7, a rare condition has emerged known as MIS-C. The condition was first identified in

Pre-existing conditions

Health issues that are already affecting an individual prior to becoming infected with a disease such as COVID-19.

the United Kingdom in April 2020 and is a unique and potentially deadly manifestation of COVID-19. (In the United Kingdom, the disorder goes by the name **pediatric inflammatory multisystem syndrome [PIMS-TS]**.) The disorder causes severe inflammation in blood vessels, the heart, lungs, eyes, and brain. The inflammation in blood vessels can lead to serious heart damage, and, in extremely rare instances, it can be fatal. Doctors do not yet know why some youngsters fall victim to the syndrome. For many children, there is no evidence of active coronavirus infection as MIS-C symptoms begin to emerge.

According to the CDC, signs and symptoms of MIS-C may include fever, abdominal pain, vomiting, diarrhea, neck pain, rash, bloodshot eyes, and fatigue. However, the CDC, Mayo Clinic, and Boston Children's Hospital advise parents that the most common symptom is a fever that lasts for more than 24 hours and may be present for several days. A child may also have symptoms that commonly occur in **Kawasaki disease**: red eyes, swollen hands, and cracked lips. Gastrointestinal distress may be another early symptom.

MIS-C is most similar to Kawasaki disease and toxic shock syndrome, but as medical investigators have begun learning more about COVID-19 in general, they are additionally gaining keener insight into MIS-C. Researchers at Evelina London Children's Hospital and King's College London have conducted a series of studies, which have shown that the syndrome not only causes extreme inflammation, but also adversely affects the immune system. In an analysis published in *Nature Medicine*, the medical investigators found that in the acute stage of MIS-C syndrome, children have elevated levels of proteins called **cytokines**, which play prominently in triggering an inflammatory assault. Children also have reduced levels of **lymphocytes**, a key population of white blood cells that are critical to the immune response. The syndrome's symptoms are unique to CO-VID-19, concluded Dr. Manu Shankar-Hari, who led the team of medical investigators. PIMS-TS, as Shankar-Hari refers to it, is a syndrome that is new to medical science: "PIMS-TS is a new syndrome. Our research has allowed us to provide the first description of the profound immune system changes in severely ill children with this new illness," Shankar-Hari said in a statement. In the acute phase of the syndrome the population of "lymphocytes, a particular type of white cell involved in specific protective immunity, are depleted," Shankar-Hari explained, noting that even as these immune cells are declining, they are still fighting SARS-CoV-2, albeit as an army, but with far fewer troops. Remarkably, when the child recovers, these important components of the immune system rebound, the research found.

Lymphocytes

White blood cells that are important in immunity.

38. Does exposure to common cold viruses help lessen the severity of COVID-19?

Some medical experts believe the reason children remain asymptomatic or experience only a mild case of COVID-19 is due to previous exposure to coronaviruses that cause the common cold. Children frequently catch colds, which tend to spread like wildfire in schools. Four distinct coronaviruses are known to cause the seasonal illness, and it is possible, some experts theorize, that children's immune systems recognize the spike proteins of other coronaviruses and develop an antibody and/or cellular immune response against them. All coronaviruses use their "spikes" to initiate infection of human cells. But while that it is a compelling theory, it is also possible that children respond differently to SARS-CoV-2 than adults, especially people 65 and older, who tend to have more debilitating bouts with the infection because of age-related immune system inefficiency. Children, some doctors contend, have a powerful innate immune response, referring to the body's frontline assault on infectious agents.

39. Are children and young adults silent spreaders of SARS-CoV-2?

If doctors at Massachusetts General Hospital are correct—and their data support this—children and college-age young people may play a more pivotal role in the community spread of SARS-CoV-2 than scientists originally thought. Children may be among the most prolific **silent spreaders** of SARS-CoV-2, the virus that causes COVID-19.

Silent spreaders

Healthy-seeming individuals who nonetheless carry a high viral load and contribute significantly to the spread of disease.

In the early months of the pandemic, it was thought children were less likely to spread SARS-CoV-2 because they were said to have fewer ACE2 receptors on their cells. ACE2 receptors, as you may recall from Question 10, are the sites that SARS-CoV-2 latches onto as it seeks to unlock and infect human cells. But the Mass General research group argues in *The Journal of Pediatrics* that even though youngsters have fewer sites to which the virus can attach, they are still capable of carrying a significant viral load in their nasal passages and throats. Children were found to have a significantly higher level of coronavirus in their airways than hospitalized adults in ICUs being treated for COVID-19. "I was surprised by the high level of virus we found in children of all ages, especially in the first two days of infection," Dr. Lael Yonker, lead author of the report, said in a statement. "I was not expecting the viral load to be so high. You think of a hospital and of all of the precautions taken to treat severely ill adults, but the viral loads of these hospitalized patients are significantly lower than [those of] a healthy child who is walking around with a high SARS-CoV-2 viral load."

40. What was the point of closing schools if kids mostly get mild or asymptomatic infections?

Closing schools is what is known in public health as a **non-pharmaceutical intervention**—that is, an intervention seeking to change the social conditions that allow virus transmission rather than attempting to prevent it through biomedical methods such as a medication or a vaccine. It has long been known that schools are risky sites for communicable diseases—the common cold and influenza spread prolifically through schools. Dozens of children are in classrooms for hours, and many buildings are old, dilapidated, and, most important, lacking in sufficient ventilation—conditions that are ripe for **aerosol transmission**. School closures are not an impulsive strategy that suddenly emerged in 2020; they have long-standing roots around the world, dating back to the era before a disease-mitigating vaccine could thwart serious childhood infections like measles and polio.

The theory behind closing schools is to interrupt the chains of transmission that can occur as a virus moves from person to person in large groups of people. It also prevents schoolchildren from carrying the pathogen home, possibly posing risks to vulnerable infant siblings, parents, and grandparents. In the CDC's study of pediatric hospitalizations, 188 of 576 children hospitalized for COVID-19 in the 14 hospitals studied between

Non-pharmaceutical intervention

A public health effort that seeks to alter people's behavior with the goal of interrupting the chain of virus transmission in large groups of people.

Aerosol transmission

Spread of disease carried via respiratory droplets transferred into the air from a cough, sneeze, or even talking or singing.

March and July of 2020 were newborns and toddlers, ages 0 to 23 months, evidence that babies have been stricken. It is impossible to say which students will have mild or asymptomatic SARS-CoV-2 infections and which ones will progress to serious COVID-19 requiring hospitalization. To err on the side of safety, schools are ordered closed to prevent infection clusters—and to ensure the safety of the most vulnerable, including children with asthma, diabetes, and rare medical conditions within the student populations of schools worldwide.

School closures are not ordered on a whim. They come about rarely and only when an infectious disease poses such a catastrophic threat to human life that leaving schools—and businesses—open would imperil the lives of many. One of the take-home messages of the COVID-19 pandemic is that schools are not populated by students alone. Obituaries emerged as early as the spring of 2020 reporting the deaths of teachers throughout the country. Deaths of teachers in Arizona, Mississippi, Texas, and beyond were among the unexpected threats of the pandemic. In New York City, teachers, a principal, and support personnel in several schools died of COVID-19, which they contracted before schools were officially ordered closed. Among those who died was Rana Zoe Mungin of Brooklyn, a 30-year-old teacher who faced obstacles in her efforts to be tested for the coronavirus. Had schools closed sooner, her life, and possibly those of others, might have been spared.

So, do closures work? To answer that, we can look at previous examples from history. School closures were among the non-pharmaceutical strategies in the United States during the pandemic of 1918–1919, which was arguably the deadliest flu season in global history. In the early 20th century, cities that closed schools and other venues early in the pandemic saved more lives of its citizens than those that waited until the virus was already spreading rapidly in their communities. A frequently cited example is the difference between how St. Louis and Philadelphia responded in 1918. St. Louis fared better than Philadelphia because interventions were implemented sooner. In September 1918, while St. Louis closed its schools, parks, churches, and other public spaces, Philadelphia allowed the massive Liberty Loan Parade to take place on September 28, 1918, an event attended by thousands. Not long after the parade, the city was stricken by one of the worst outbreaks in the country.

School closures have been used in more recent history, too. In the H1N1 influenza pandemic of 2009, schools were advised by the CDC to close for two weeks during the pandemic's spring wave in April and May. At that time, 700 schools across the country ceased classes as the novel H1N1 flu strain circulated. Among the closures were 50 schools in New York City, where an estimated 800,000 residents were stricken with H1N1 flu. The CDC, however, reversed its guidance the following August, recommending that schools should not close unless local health officials were aware of elevated rates of infection in their communities. Dr. Thomas Frieden, director of the CDC in 2009, said additional data compiled on H1N1's behavior after the spring wave made school closings a matter of local choice.

In the early 20th century, cities that closed schools and other venues early in the pandemic saved more lives of its citizens than those that waited until the virus was already spreading rapidly in their communities.

41. Is there a way to open schools safely during a pandemic?

In South Korea, children work at desks that are surrounded on three sides by a plexiglass shield. They wear face masks and have their temperatures monitored twice daily. These protective measures could become the model of how to operate schools in a pandemic. Yoosun Yun and colleagues of Samsung Medical Center in Seoul have been tracking how students progressed following the reopening of schools as lockdown measures were eased throughout the country. The key to successful reopenings, according to the Samsung investigators, is to resume in-person classes when community spread of SARS-CoV-2 is low.

Children in South Korea went back to school when infections fell below 50 new coronavirus cases daily, which Smriti Mallapaty, reporting in the journal *Nature*, estimated to be "equivalent to 1 case per million people."

On the flip side, when community transmission is high, reopening schools risks clusters and outbreaks of SARS-CoV-2, because infections among students reflect the burden of disease in the community as a whole. Shortly after starting the academic year in August 2020, the University of North Carolina at Chapel Hill and the University of Notre Dame, among others, were forced to switch to virtual classes because the elevated transmission rate of the virus on campus made in-person classes too risky. Other universities stayed open, only to experience significant outbreaks: in late August, the University of Alabama had over 500 cases, the University of Missouri had 160, and Iowa State had 130.

42. What can preschools do to prevent the spread of SARS-CoV-2 infection?

As K–12 schools debated reopening in the midst of a pandemic throughout the United States, directors of preschools in major cities reopened without much fanfare or discussion. Why?

Preschools are considered essential businesses in many states. California is no exception.

Dr. Stephanie Taylor-Dinwiddie, executive director of Spirit Child Development Center in Los Angeles, said her center closed when a COVID-19 State of Emergency was declared in California in March of 2020. The center reopened in June, however, to meet the needs of parents. The pandemic didn't wane in California the way it did in New York, but expanded to such an extent that California ultimately became the state with the highest number of coronavirus cases in the country.

Like her counterparts in other major cities, reopening meant following state health department and federal guidelines on masks, physical distancing, and hand hygiene. She also altered the way meals are served to strengthen safety measures. "We previously practiced family-style meal service where children learned how to serve themselves from central bowls and platters that were placed in the middle of the table," Taylor-Dinwiddie said. "This practice has been discontinued for the foreseeable future."

Changes have additionally meant a crash course for 3- and 4-year-olds on the principles of infection control. Reopening was important, Taylor-Dinwiddie said, because a significant number of her center's students are the children of essential workers. "We have a mix of families in our center," Taylor-Dinwiddie said. "Some of our parents are considered essential workers, which includes health care, restaurant workers, the clergy, maintenance personnel, and company executives."

To mitigate potential infection, children must wear masks at all times except for meals. "When a child arrives we take their temperature. If a temperature reading is 100.4[°F] or above, the child is not allowed entry. If the child has a cough, entry is not allowed." Runny noses can also bar entry unless the child's physician confirms the symptom is the result of allergies. "Our classrooms have been reconfigured into learning pods that are spaced 6 feet apart to allow social distancing. Instead of children having the benefit of multiple teachers, our teachers are assigned a smaller group of children to work with exclusively."

Everyone wears a mask, which reinforces mask-wearing among the children. Teachers additionally wear face shields. In the era before COVID-19, parents were allowed in the school. Now, even parents must be masked and come no farther than the entry.

43. Can SARS-CoV-2 be transmitted in the food or beverages that my child consumes?

There is "no evidence" that SARS-CoV-2 can be transmitted through food, said Dr. Mike Ryan, executive director of the World Health Organization's emergencies program, during a news conference in August 2020. His words of assurance came after concerns were raised in China. Reports in three Chinese cities have claimed the virus was detected on the surface of imported frozen food. The claims inspired Chinese health officials to launch an investigation to determine if the alleged discovery is genuine. The CDC has remained steadfast in its stance that SARS-CoV-2 cannot be transmitted through the food supply.

PART FIVE

Coronavirus Infection: Immunity, Aging, and Disease Spread

What basics should I know about the immune system?

What is the adaptive immune system, and why is it important?

How serious is COVID-19 for people 65 and older?

More . . .

Immune system

The network of cells, proteins, and organs that protects and heals the body from infection, injury, and dysfunction.

Immunologists

Scientists and physicians who specialize in studying the immune system.

Innate immune system

Protective barriers, such as the skin, as well as immune cells, and secretions present at birth that protect the body from infection.

Adaptive immune system

Immunity not present at birth that develops over time as a result of exposure to pathogens.

Barrier tissues

Tissues that present a physical blockade to pathogens, such as skin or mucous membranes.

Mucus

A secretion that traps pathogenic microbes to prevent them from entering the body.

44. What basics should I know about the immune system?

The **immune system** is the body's defense system, one of the most complex networks of surveillance and protection in the known universe. Nothing human-made comes close. Indeed, the human immune system is so complex that **immunologists** say they've learned only a portion of what remains to be understood. It is a system so precise that it detects viruses measuring only nanometers in size, and so keen that vaccine doses are administered in mere micrograms.

Our intricate network of protection shields us against an otherwise hostile world through a double-pronged defense: an **innate immune system**, which is present at birth and continues throughout life, and an **adaptive immune system** (also known as acquired immunity) that develops over time. Some critical adaptive immune responses decline as people reach advanced ages. Innate immunity remains roughly intact.

The innate system is made up of **barrier tissues**, such as the skin and mucosal membranes, which form physical blockades to keep pathogens from entering. Mucosal membranes secrete **mucus**, a substance that further discourages the invasion of pathogens.

When viruses, bacteria, or fungi do invade, the innate immune system has a broad array of responses, which run the gamut from cells that eat the invaders to those that secrete **proinflammatory molecules** that cause tissues to swell and signals to be sent, marshaling more forces to destroy the invader. Sometimes, in the course of enemy annihilation, this cascade of inflammatory molecules harms healthy tissue, something we'll discuss in Question 46. Innate immunity is made up of white blood cells or leukocytes; some move freely throughout the body eliminating cellular debris, while others are largely residents of certain tissues and are therefore less mobile. All white blood cells begin their lives in the bone marrow and are derived from **stem cells**—cells that are blank slates, capable of morphing into any one of many types of blood cells.

Members of the innate immune system include a long roster of cells, many of which perform more than one duty. **Granulocytes** are cells such as neutrophils, eosinophils, basophils, and mast cells. One of their main roles is to identify and annihilate pathogenic invaders. They're called granulocytes because they secrete **granules**, which are compounds that cause damage to pathogens.

For example, **neutrophils** are highly abundant and mobile but short-lived white blood cells that secrete primary and secondary granules. Some of the primary granules include antibacterial compounds known as acid hydrolases and defensins. Secondary granules are among the most abundant because they activate the system called complement, more formally referred to as the **complement cascade**. The complement system is a series of sequential activities that mark pathogens for destruction by immune system cells. One way this destruction occurs is by a process called **phagocytosis**—the word means "ingesting or eating infiltrators," which is a major function of white cells that are phagocytes. **Macrophages** (the name literally means "big eaters") are the largest of all white blood cells and the biggest eaters, but they are not the most abundant. Neutrophils, which in addition to producing granules are also phagocytic, are the most abundant white cells.

The ranks of white blood cells of the innate immune system include several other members: Dendritic, natural killer, and tissue-resident lymphoid cells, all members of the white blood cell army.

Proinflammatory molecules

Cells that are blank slates, capable of morphing into any one of many types of blood cells.

Leukocytes

Any of a number of white blood cells that fight disease and repair damaged tissues.

Stem cells

Undifferentiated cells that have the capacity to develop into any type of cell needed.

Granulocytes

Immune cells that secrete granules to destroy invading microbes.

Granules

Chemical compounds produced by immune cells that defend against or identify invasive microbes.

Neutrophils

Highly abundant and mobile but short-lived white blood cells that secrete primary and secondary granules.

Complement cascade

A series of sequential activities that mark pathogens for destruction by other immune cells.

Phagocytosis

The process of engulfing and destroying pathogenic infiltrators.

Macrophages

Large white blood cells that have the task of destroying pathogens by phagocytosis.

Pathogen-associated molecular patterns (PAMPs)

A set of general characteristics that the innate system uses to identify invasive microbes.

Hypochlorite

A chemical produced by immune cells that kills invading microbes.

The innate immune system is known for its rapid response, and, in terms of evolution, it is the oldest form of immunity. Most people live lengthy lives and never realize the extent of the wars that have been waged in their own bodies, battles launched by the innate immune system against countless infiltrators. Unlike the adaptive immune response, which is a more precise approach that produces a targeted response to a specific invasive threat, the innate system is on patrol in search of invaders based on generalized patterns called **pathogen-associated molecular patterns** (PAMPs). Among these patterns are the complex structures on the surfaces of bacteria, or the genetic material of viruses, such as their RNA or DNA, depending on the genetic material with which the virus is endowed. SARS-CoV-2 and all its relatives in the coronavirus family are RNA viruses.

Throughout a person's life, the innate immune response is the body's first line of defense, capable of responding to invasive threats and bodily injury. In the event of a novel viral infection, such as a pandemic virus, the innate immune system spares none of its troops or any of its activities—all can be unleashed with explosive ferocity, including a SWAT team known in cell biology as the professional phagocytes. These innate immune system cells seek out infiltrators and gobble them up. Phagocytosis is the process of engulfing and destroying pathogenic infiltrators. Even if these cells just ate their enemies and did nothing more, it seems that activity alone would be enough. But once an enemy is engulfed, phagocytes unleash a chemical attack. To finish off the enemy, phagocytes release within themselves a blast of **hypochlorite** (which is a key component of the disinfectant we call "bleach") along a shower of other harsh compounds. Professional phagocytes are made up of the large cells known as macrophages as well as the smaller neutrophils, also called polymorphs.

In the 19th century, Russian zoologist Elie Metchnikoff concluded that phagocytosis formed the main defense against infection. As brilliant as Metchnikoff was, it turns out that he was wrong. From a 21st-century vantage point, immunologists now know the innate immune system is far more complex, yet lacks the specificity of adaptive immunity. The innate immune system also releases pro-inflammatory molecules that ramp up **inflammation**—something you've probably experienced, but may not know exactly what's going on. Nature designed the inflammatory response as a powerful form of protection: blood vessels in the infected area dilate and the temperature rises causing the skin to redden and affected tissues to swell. These activities help speed up the ability of immune cells to reach the infection, remove invaders and start the healing process.

Unfortunately, when faced with a pandemic virus like SARS-CoV-2, the innate response can be especially furious in some people—it isn't easily switched off in severe COVID-19. Many cells of the innate system can increase the inflammatory response: macrophages, for example, secrete proteins that prompt the recruitment more pro-inflammatory cells and molecules from the blood. Mast cells release floods of cytokines. In severe COVID-19, this explosive cascade of cytokines, **chemokines**, **histamine**, and other pro-inflammatory molecules results in a betrayal of the patient's own healthy organs and tissues. The inflammation that occurs in severe COVID-19 can cause tissue damage as a direct consequence of the innate immune system's aggression. For people with severe COVID-19, an extreme cytokine response is often referred to as a **cytokine storm**,

Inflammation

An immune response that triggers a set of physical and chemical reactions focused toward eliminating the threat, removing damaged tissue, and healing the affected area.

Chemokines

Proteins released by immune cells that attract other immune cells to the site of an injury or infection.

Histamine

A chemical produced by granulocytes that triggers inflammation in response to an injury or antigen.

Cytokine storm

An extreme innate immune release of cytokines that can be harmful or even fatal.

an innate immune system response that, in some instances, can prove fatal.

In September 2020, the World Health Organization updated its guidelines on how best to respond pharmaceutically to severe COVID-19. The agency recommends corticosteroid medications, like dexamethasone, as the treatment of choice for advanced COVID-19. Corticosteroid medications work to reduce the inflammatory response so that it doesn't overwhelm the body; some of these medications are used in treating common inflammatory disorders, such as asthma, eczema, and other inflammatory disorders. In an editorial in the *Journal of the American Medical Association* (*JAMA*) that accompanied four studies on corticosteroids used for treating COVID-19, Dr. Hallie Prescott of the University of Michigan, Ann Arbor and Dr. Todd Rice of Vanderbilt University in Tennessee declared that the research represented "a step forward" in the treatment of critically ill patients with COVID-19.

The innate immune system may be defending the front lines, but it can also call for backup. Dendritic cells, innate immune cells roughly resembling microscopic starfish that can phagocytose invaders, also have another, equally important role: They summon the adaptive immune system to get a move on and help knock out the infection. Dendritic cells use their "arms" to grab a few fragments from the damaged enemy under attack and present them to adaptive immune cells called T cells. These cells will be discussed further in Questions 47 and 49, but for now it's enough to know that T cells are experts at killing entire virus-infected cells. The key point to learn from this example, though, is that the innate and the adaptive immune systems collaborate in their efforts to extinguish an infiltrator.

45. What are cytokines, and what do they do?

The term "cytokine" is a general name for an array of dynamic proteins: chemokines, interferons, interleukins, and tumor necrosis factors. They may seem confusing because their complex activities are often very similar. In other words, there is a significant degree of redundancy in their functions. These infinitesimal proteins can be further defined as signaling molecules that are involved in nearby and long-distance communications between cells. Most important, they mediate the immune response by triggering specific activities in response to infiltrators. To develop a stronger grasp of these proteins it's a good idea to understand how they are grouped. For example, lymphokines are cytokines produced by lymphocytes; monokines are made by monocytes; interleukins are produced by leukocytes and act on other leukocytes; chemokines are cytokines that have chemotactic activity, which means these cytokines can move macrophages and neutrophils to sites of infection.

Nature endowed the immune system with cytokines that are **pro-inflammatory** as well as those that are **anti-inflammatory**. All are secreted by diverse populations of immune system cells. Inflammation is important in a healthy response to viral infection because it is part of a broad response to ridding the body of a potentially deadly invader. Hallmarks of inflammation are swelling of affected tissues, a rise in their temperature, and a spike in pain throughout the affected region.

Pro-inflammatory cytokine

A type of signaling molecule (a cytokine) that is secreted from immune cells like helper T cells (Th) and macrophages, and certain other cell types that promote inflammation.

Anti-inflammatory

A series of immunoregulatory molecules that control the pro-inflammatory cytokine response.

One of the first cytokines to arrive at a site of viral infection is tumor necrosis factor-alpha (TNF-α), which is released by macrophages and monocytes. TNF-α binds to infected cells to initiate antiviral activities to prevent viral spread. Other pro-inflammatory cytokines include interferon-gamma, a variety of chemokines, and various interleukins.

Cytokines are not the only pro-inflammatory molecules. Histamine, which is stored in the granules of mast cells and basophils, can act as a powerful inflammatory molecule. It is released from these cells during the stimuli generated by acute inflammation.

46. How do cytokines and other immune components cause severe COVID-19?

For many people, the innate immune response can completely knock out infections, including mild infections of COVID-19, without the need for added fire power from the adaptive immune system. But that isn't the story for everyone with COVID-19 because the innate response can lose its coordinated synchrony, its timing can be thrown off as it attempts to fight a pandemic virus, a menace that is equipped with an array of wily tricks to help it outfox the innate immune system. In severe COVID-19, medical scientists are keenly aware that the immune response becomes dysregulated and loses the ability to slam on the brakes.

Dr. Matthew Woodruff, an immunologist at the Lowance Center for Human Immunology at Emory University, says preventing a dysregulated immune response may be as important as treating the virus itself.

This is why dexamethasone has become an important medication in the treatment of severe COVID-19. Woodruff and his Emory colleagues in the laboratory of Dr. Ignacio Sanz report that even though severe COVID-19 is an infectious disease, it has potent features of an **autoimmune condition**. The body is at war with itself as components of the immune system— pro-inflammatory molecules, antibodies, and lymphocytes—explosively emerge as turncoats, assaulting otherwise healthy organs and tissues. Woodruff underscores that the presence of rogue antibodies is an integral part of the overall attack. "In patients with severe COVID-19 infections, evidence emerged that the inflammatory processes used to fight the SARS-CoV-2 virus were, in addition to fighting the virus, responsible for harming the patient. Clinical studies described cytokine storms in which the immune system produced an overwhelming quantity of inflammatory molecules, antibodies triggering dangerous blood clots, and inflammation of multiple organ systems," Woodruff wrote in the online publication, *The Conversation*.

Precisely why the immune system goes awry in COVID-19 remains an ongoing subject of debate. In the journal *Science*, Dr. Jamie Garfield, a pulmonologist at Temple University Hospital argued that hyperinflammatory responses are a major problem in the care of patients with severe COVID-19. "The real morbidity and mortality of this disease is probably driven by this out of proportion inflammatory response to the virus," Garfield said.

In the same report, Dr. Joseph Levitt, a pulmonary critical physician at Stanford University School of Medicine argued to the contrary: "There seems to have been a quick move to associate COVID-19 with these

Autoimmune condition

An autoimmune disease is a condition in which your immune system mistakenly attacks your body. The immune system normally guards against germs like bacteria and viruses. When it senses these foreign invaders, it sends out an army of fighter cells to attack them.

hyperinflammatory states. I haven't really seen convincing data that that is the case."

An estimated 15% of all COVID cases are considered severe, the majority characterized by substantial to critical inflammation in the lungs requiring supplemental oxygen. Doctors have additionally detected abnormal blood clotting among a constellation of problems in patients with severe disease. An estimated 5% of severe COVID-19 patients require treatment with a ventilator. Meanwhile, a type of COVID-related hyperinflammatory state in adults emerged in the summer of 2020 (Question 53), which resembles multisystem inflammatory syndrome in children (MIS-C). The condition was detected in patients in the United States and abroad. It is characterized by severe inflammation resembling toxic shock syndrome. What makes it unique and a standalone diagnosis, according to the CDC, is the absence of inflammation in the lungs.

47. What is the adaptive immune system, and why is it important?

B lymphocytes

Lymphocytes that provide the "record-keeping" or memory function of the adaptive immune system.

T lymphocytes

White blood cells also known as T cells. They are members of the adaptive immune system and fight invasive infectious agents, including viruses, and also play a role in targeting cancer cells.

Just as the innate immune system is known for its rapid but generalized immune response, the adaptive system is about specificity—making sure the response is tailored to the exact pathogen being encountered. The adaptive immune system is like a biological computer that uses data-driven activities, such as forming a memory of every infection—major and minor—to help keep the body healthy throughout life.

The adaptive immune system is the powerful cellular-based system that relies on two broad categories of white blood cells: **B lymphocytes** and **T lymphocytes**, commonly referred to as B cells and T cells. A specific type of B cell, called a plasma cell, produces antibodies (see Question 49). Specific types of T cells can target infections that have invaded the body's cells and destroy those that are afflicted. T cells also target and destroy cells invaded by cancer.

As with cells of the innate immune system, those in the adaptive immune system also begin their lives in the bone marrow. Both B and T cells are derived from a type of stem cell known as multipotent hematopoietic stem cells, but they follow very different paths once they start to develop. The "B" of B cells refers to the word "bone," because B cells form and mature in the bone marrow, emerging out of the marrow as **naïve B cells**. Naïve B cells migrate out of the bone marrow, circulating through the lymphatic system. **Precursor T lymphocytes**, on the other hand, emerge from the marrow and migrate to the **thymus gland**—a small gland located behind your sternum and just below your collarbone (not to be confused with the thyroid gland, which is in your throat). The fact that they mature in the thymus is why they're called T cells, as the "T" comes from the first letter of thymus. While in the gland, T cells develop T-cell receptors (TCRs) and other special receptors known as CD4 and CD8.

Adaptive immunity isn't present at birth and generally doesn't start recognizing and mounting a response against foreign infiltrators until 6 to 9 months of age. This form of protection forms over many years, and while it interacts with the innate system to rid the body of threats, the adaptive system also maintains stunning recall—a memory—of previous infections. Adaptive immunity is exploited to form memories based on the infinitesimal substances introduced through vaccination, immunizing us against deadly threats. Most amazing, though, is the specificity of the adaptive system, which not only retains a

Naïve B cells

B cells that have just emerged from the bone marrow and not yet encountered a pathogen.

Precursor T lymphocytes

Developing T cells that have emerged from the bone marrow; these migrate to the thymus gland to finish their development.

Thymus gland

A small gland behind the sternum that houses maturing T cells.

memory of an infectious agent, but when it "sees" it again, launches a battalion of neutralizing antibodies and cellular soldiers. The memory of some infections is lifelong.

For example, most people born in the United States before 1957 are immune to measles, not because of vaccination but because of natural infection. The adaptive immune system created antibodies specific to the virus and additionally developed an indelible memory of the threat. As a result of having dealt with an infiltrator in the past, the adaptive response is accelerated and more robust when the infectious agent is encountered in the future.

The reason a new pandemic virus such as SARS-CoV-2 can pose a problem for the adaptive immune system is because it has no record of the offending pathogen—so it doesn't know that it should respond. We know that some people were able to shake off the infection after a mild to moderate illness, but others had to be hospitalized and admitted to an intensive care unit for weeks, and tens of thousands of people died. Still others who were hospitalized and eventually released reported residual physiological problems that ranged from headaches to breathing disturbances and fatigue that continued for months after discharge.

48. What are T cells, and what do they do?

Cytotoxic T cells

An important population of T lymphocytes because these cells can kill cells that have been infected with viruses, including any type of coronavirus.

There are four types of T cells that are prominent in adaptive immunity: cytotoxic, helper, memory, and regulatory. We'll take a look at each type in turn.

- **Cytotoxic T cells** are an important population of T lymphocytes because these cells can kill cells that have been infected with viruses, including any type of coronavirus. A cytotoxic T cell is also known as "cytotoxic T lymphocyte," CD8+ T cell, or by the blunter nickname of "killer T cell."

- **Helper T cells** are sometimes called the most important cells in adaptive immunity. This population of T cells is critical for most adaptive and some innate immune system responses. For example, they are required for proper functioning of the B cell response by helping B cells secrete antibodies (see Question 47). Helper T cells also aid macrophages in the annihilation of ingested pathogens and play a critical role in the function of cytotoxic T cells' ability to kill targeted infected or cancerous cells.

- **Memory T cells** recall a past infection and produce an accelerated and more robust response to reinfection. Vaccination relies on memory T cells to recall exposure to specific antigens and to set immune responses in motion to ensure that the pathogen does not cause reinfection.

- **Regulatory T cells** were at one time known as suppressor T cells. They play a role in quieting the immune system. For example, regulatory T cells secrete anti-inflammatory cytokines to regulate immune function and prevent the immune system from attacking the body's own tissues (autoimmunity). Mature regulatory T cells can carry surface proteins, such as CD4, FOXP3, and CD25. The main role of regulatory T cells, which are known by the shorthand, Tregs, is preventing autoimmune diseases and limiting conditions caused by chronic inflammation.

There is also a unique population referred to as gamma-delta ($\gamma\delta$) T cells, sometimes referred to as "unconventional" T cells. This population represents a small subset of lymphocytes, but recent studies suggest that they primarily play an important role in the lungs.

Helper T cells

These cells are critical for most adaptive and some innate immune system responses.

Memory T cells

Antigen-specific T cells that remain long-term after an infection has been eliminated.

Regulatory T cells

These cells play a role in quieting the immune system.

49. How important are B cells?

B cells are as important in the adaptive immune system as T cells. They help fight bacteria and viruses and are not subject to decline, as is the case with T cells. B cells can be found in the spleen, lymph nodes, and tonsils, and there are three types that are important to know. Naïve B cells, as discussed in Question 47, are those that have not been exposed to an antigen (a fragment of an infectious agent, for example, such as a virus or bacterium) and therefore can be thought of as soldiers waiting for an assignment. The other two key active B cells that are important to know are **plasma cells**, also called effector B cells, which are responsible for producing antibodies, and **memory B cells**, which can survive for decades. Memory B cells are found in the so-called germinal centers of the lymph nodes and spleen; they begin as naïve B cells but are activated when infection occurs and a helper T cell presents an antigen to the memory B cell. Upon reinfection, a memory B cell that already has a record of the pathogen produces an accelerated, robust response against the infectious agent. Memory B cells can also differentiate into plasma B cells, especially in the event of reinfection, to produce the first flood of antibodies to help wipe out the infiltrator.

Plasma cell

A specific form of B cell that produces antibodies.

Memory B cell

A B cell that retains a long-term memory of pathogens encountered in the past.

50. How important are antibodies?

Antibodies are produced by plasma (effector B cells) and are among the most vital components in the adaptive immune system. Antibodies, also referred to as **immunoglobulins** (abbreviated as Ig), are a family of five proteins. Each type—or isoform, as they are formally known—plays a specific role in the adaptive immune response. These five proteins are called IgM, IgG, IgA, IgE, and IgD.

- **IgM** is the largest antibody and the first type to be secreted in response to a pathogen. It is the only

Antibodies

A complex family of proteins that plays a specific role in the adaptive immune response.

Immunoglobulin

Any of the five proteins that make up human antibodies: IgM, IgG, IgA, IgE, and IgD.

immunoglobulin that has a pentameric (meaning five arms) shape, making it look somewhat like a star; the other antibodies have only two arms, giving them the appearance of the letter "Y." IgM is produced as soon as an antigen is recognized and is a neutralizing antibody. It swarms straight to the infection site but is relatively transient, because its job is to send signals to initiate the production of IgG.

- **IgG** accounts for about 75% of all the immunoglobulins in human blood. It is produced in four subgroups: IgG1, IgG2, IgG3, and IgG4. On the whole, it is extremely versatile, triggering phagocytosis and initiating the antibody-dependent cell-mediated cytotoxicity response.

- **IgA** is found in mucus, saliva, breast milk, serum, and intestinal fluid. As with IgG, there are subtypes, but only two: IgA1 and IgA2, which have molecular differences. This is the immunoglobulin that is found on mucosal surfaces (like the insides of your nose and mouth) and defends against inhaled pathogens.

- Among immunoglobulins, **IgE** is detected the least frequently. It is important in allergies and parasitic infections.

- **IgD** largely functions as a receptor on B cells and may be involved in the B-cell maturation process and other vital B-cell roles.

51. How serious is COVID-19 for people 65 and older?

One of the first challenges in a pandemic is to identify segments of the population at highest risk of morbidity and mortality and to institute measures to shield these people as much as possible from infection. You may be familiar with efforts to protect residents of congregate living facilities, such as nursing homes, which barred visitors to block potential coronavirus carriers from entering. Early mandates for masks were for older people and anyone with a chronic medical condition. Older populations have been especially vulnerable to COVID-19, which is one reason this population was prioritized for COVID-19 vaccinations.

Although people of all ages have developed the infection and have died of the disease, it is clear that those who have borne the brunt of the pandemic virus have been the oldest.

Age is the consistent risk factor for severe COVID-19 in every country around the globe. The CDC estimates that out of every 10 deaths related to COVID-19 in the United States, eight involve people 65 and older. The agency also calculates risk as increasing with each decade of life. In other words, people in their 50s are at higher risk of COVID-19 complications requiring hospitalization than people in their 40s. By the same token, people in their 60s are higher risk than those in their 50s, and so on.

The body becomes less efficient at fighting new infections with age.

A study reported in the July 2020 issue of the journal *Nature* found that COVID-19 patients who were older than 80 were about 20 times more likely to die of the infection than people in their 50s. In New York City, which had one of the worst outbreaks nationwide, nearly half of all COVID-19 deaths occurred among people 75 or older. What this says about the adaptive immune system is instructive: The body becomes less efficient at fighting new infections with increasing age.

This loss of efficiency occurs largely among T cells and with the thymus gland itself. The thymus gland ungergoes its most robust growth in very early childhood, but it declines gradually, starting at age 20 and possibly even earlier. Total **thymic involution**, a condition in which the glandular tissue has been replaced by fat, usually is evident around age 60, which means from that time onward, we do not make new T cells. The key characteristic of thymic involution is shrinkage of the gland and loss of its architectural shape. This loss explains the increase in infectious disease susceptibility in older populations and the increase in cancer susceptibility as well. However, there are reports of T cell maturation in the liver and intestines after the thymus gland declines.

Thymic involution

A condition in older adults in which thymus gland tissue has been replaced by fat, such that the person no longer makes new T cells in the thymus.

Along with the specific age-related probability of COVID-19 complications, the risk of illness requiring hospitalization increases with age in general. There is a greater preponderance of underlying medical conditions, or **comorbidities**, which often occur as people age. Older people are more likely than younger ones to have diabetes, coronary artery disease, heart failure, chronic obstructive pulmonary disease (COPD), and other respiratory problems. Obesity has been shown to be a **risk factor** for severe COVID-19, regardless of age. Even among children, excess weight exacerbates the potential for complications. Comorbidities can complicate COVID-19 and increase the risk of death.

Comorbidities

Underlying medical conditions that can complicate the progress of a newly acquired illness.

Risk factor

A specific condition or situation that increases a person's risk of disease or poor disease outcomes.

52. Why does the immune system decline with age?

As powerful as the system is—capable of thwarting threats over many decades—it doesn't remain robust throughout life. It declines with age, which means your body may not mount as vigorous a response to infections as it did when you were younger. Medical scientists refer to this phenomenon as **immune senescence**, which basically means aging of the immune system.

Immune senescence explains why the virus that causes chickenpox in childhood—varicella zoster—can rebound, as an excruciatingly painful bout with shingles starting around age 60, or sometimes sooner. The virus never really goes away but remains dormant as a result of suppression by a healthy immune system.

The overall decline in immunity with age predisposes older adults to a higher risk of acute viral and bacterial infections in general. Hospital-acquired infections, for example, have their greatest impact on older patients, and studies have shown that mortality rates resulting from these infections are three times higher among older adults than for younger individuals. The increased risk for greater mortality is due to impaired adaptive immunity in older populations.

53. Is there a condition in adults that is comparable to MIS-C in children?

Since the spring of 2020, physicians in the United States and the United Kingdom have been aware of a serious pediatric condition that is unique to COVID-19, called multisystem inflammatory syndrome (see Questions 7 and 37). By late summer, medical investigators began studying a comparable condition in adults typified by cardiovascular, gastrointestinal, dermatologic, and neurologic symptoms and accompanied by hyperinflammatory activity. The CDC has dubbed the condition multisystem inflammatory syndrome in adults (MIS-A). It is a

Immune senescence

The decreased response to infection related to the aging of the immune system.

condition that is considered new to medicine, having emerged as a COVID-related inflammatory disorder. Just as the comparable syndrome in children is characterized by a toxic shock-like condition, the same is true among adults. The CDC reported the first small cohort of adult cases in the October 2, 2020 online edition of *Morbidity and Mortality Weekly Report,* an agency publication. MIS-A typically has high levels of inflammatory markers in the blood, such as C-reactive protein and interleukin-6, among others. MIS-A is not a condition unique to older adults, but can occur in adults of any age. It is noted in this section of the book because it is a noteworthy hyper-inflammatory disorder.

The CDC learned about the condition following a number of reports submitted to the agency by health departments, doctors treating COVID-19 patients, and published case studies. What makes it different from other COVID-19-linked inflammatory conditions is the absence of pneumonia and other respiratory problems.

54. Does herd immunity protect people who are 65 and older?

Herd immunity is a simple concept that unfortunately became distorted in the early months of the COVID-19 pandemic. Herd immunity occurs when the majority of people in a community are resistant to a contagious disease. When thousands of people in a community—the herd—are resistant to diphtheria, for example, vulnerable people are protected because the disease is not being transmitted. A primary aim of herd immunity is to protect those at greatest risk of disability or death from the contagion—usually older adults and infants, but also those with impaired immunity, such as cancer patients or people with HIV. In the case of COVID-19, older adults represent the population with the highest morbidity and mortality.

Herd immunity is achieved through vaccination (see Question 24). It not brought about through widespread natural infection in communities as several armchair epidemiologists, talk radio hosts, and members of the Trump administration suggested.

Yet, even though vaccination is key, several leading scientists, including Dr. Anthony Fauci, director of the National Institute of Allergy and Infectious Diseases, doubt that the available COVID-19 vaccines will lead to herd immunity in the United States, even though vaccination may protect or partially protect individuals from infection.

Herd immunity may be an elusive goal because a significant portion of the population has vowed not to get vaccinated. Various national polls have shown that about one-third of Americans (other polls have revealed even higher fractions) are opposed to being vaccinated against COVID-19. Many of these people are vaccine skeptics—anti-vaxxers—who shun vaccines of all kinds for themselves and their children.

So where exactly does widespread natural infection stand as a public health strategy?

Nowhere, contend experts, such as Dr. Stuart Ray, a professor of medicine at the Johns Hopkins University School of Medicine. A core tenet in this belief is to abandon conventional public health strategies that are recommended to protect people from pandemic viruses—masks, social distancing, lockdowns, and school and business closures. This idea has several problems. Again, herd immunity is produced through vaccination, not by exposing people to illness. Second, young people may be at *lower* risk, but that's not the same as *no* risk; having scores of young people coming down with the infection risks killing untold numbers of them. It's worth pointing out that even if only 0.001% of children die of COVID-19, with about 73 million children under 18 in the United States, that potentially translates to over 73,000 deaths! Worse, as discussed elsewhere in the book, even children with a mild case can pass the illness to parents and grandparents, for whom the infection may prove fatal. "It's a shaky foundation on which to base a disease fighting strategy," Ray said.

55. Do coronaviruses that cause the common cold trigger seasonal infections in older adults?

Three of the four known coronaviruses that cause the common cold have been implicated as significant triggers of the seasonal illness in older adults. These three coronaviruses have been identified as OC43, NL63, and 229E (see Question 4). Together, this trio is associated with about 15% of common cold illnesses in older adults. Scientific data on these viruses as causes of common colds in people 65 and older dates back more than 20 years, preceding the discovery of all three of the more dangerous coronaviruses that emerged unexpectedly in 21st century.

The difference between infection with OC43, NL63, and 229E in younger populations and frail older people is the association with serious pneumonia. Each of these viruses can cause debilitating pneumonia in older people, especially among those with COPD and other lung conditions. The implications of this are concerning when it comes to COVID-19: If a lesser relative of SARS-CoV-2 can cause life-threatening pneumonia in an older person, but afflict a younger individual with a mere case of sniffles, just imagine how much more dangerous COVID-19 can be for that older adult—especially if it comes around seasonally, as the milder coronaviruses do.

56. Why are nursing home residents at such high risk of COVID-19?

Residents of long-term care facilities make up less than 1% of the U.S. population, but by the summer of 2020 they were estimated to constitute 41% of all U.S. COVID-19 fatalities, according to data from the CDC. There are 15,600 nursing homes in the United States, accommodating a population of approximately 1.3 million to 1.5 million people. An additional 800,000 people are residents of assisted living facilities, according to data from the American Health Care Association and the National Center for Assisted Living. The difference between the two types of congregate care are the services offered by each category. Nursing homes offer 24-hour care and monitoring. Residents of assisted living facilities require custodial care, such as help with activities of daily living.

Regardless of the type of facility, residents of both forms of congregate care were at the top of the list for COVID-19 vaccinations that began in December of 2020 and expanded the following month. The government's priority list for vaccinations included health care providers of all ages, elderly residents in congregate care and staff members of these facilities. Two messenger-RNA (mRNA) vaccines were approved by the U.S. Food and Drug

Administration in late 2020. The vaccines were found to be safe in older populations. Residents of congregate living facilities were deemed a high priority population because of their extraordinarily high COVID mortality.

COVID-19 became easily transmitted in these facilities for the same reasons that the flu, norovirus, and fast-spreading drug-resistant bacteria and fungi also have been transmitted among long-term care residents: Nursing homes and other congregate care institutions are populated with older, medically frail people. About 16.5% of U.S. long-term care residents are age 65 to 74; 26.4% are 75 to 84, and 7.8% are 95 and older.

Opportunities for exposure to SARS-CoV-2 became common in congregate living environments throughout the United States, and elsewhere globally, despite mitigation efforts. Deaths not only were high in these facilities during the early months of the pandemic, but remained elevated well into the latter months of 2020, despite masks and other measures, the CDC reported in a January, 2021 study. Even though residents are a priority population for the vaccine, doctors still do not have definitive evidence confirming how long immunity lasts. Dr. Paul Offit, a member of the FDA panel that reviewed and recommended approval the two mRNA vaccines, estimates that immunity may last for a few years. Offit is also director of the Vaccine Education Center at the University of Pennsylvania and among the leading experts who say that vaccination is needed in a broad swath of the population to achieve herd immunity.

There is no question among physicians why elderly residents of congregate living facilities needed to be at the head of the line for vaccinations. The first U.S. evidence that COVID-19 had become a deadly menace in long-term care facilities emerged in the Pacific Northwest. Nursing homes in Washington reported COVID-19 outbreaks as early as February, 2020. State public health officials quickly enacted a series of guidelines that restricted visitors and put a number of infection control measures in place. But the concerns that were initially described in Washington quickly became problems for nursing homes around the world.

Efficient nosocomial infectious agent

A pathogen that spreads in healthcare facilities.

Some scientists have referred to the virus that causes COVID-19 as an **efficient nosocomial infectious agent,** which means that it's a pathogen that spreads in healthcare facilities.

Researchers at the Centre for Evidence-Based Medicine (CEBM), an organization affiliated with the University of Oxford in the United Kingdom, have investigated COVID-19 as a nosocomial infection. A CEBM team identified hospitals, nursing homes, and dormitories as congregate living sites at risk of COVID-19 transmission.

Not only are strict infection control measures needed to prevent the spread of COVID-19, but classic methods of investigation and interviewing are required to reconstruct how the transmission started. CEBM's research builds on studies conducted in China, which also has identified the novel coronavirus as a nosocomial agent.

57. Were cruise ships vulnerable to COVID-19 outbreaks because passengers tend to be older?

While not everyone on cruise ships is older, the industry does cater to an older demographic, and, for years, these vessels have been the sites of infectious disease outbreaks that have seeded easily for several reasons: A closed environment; travelers from multiple countries; and transfers among crew members from one ship to another. The industry may require evidence of CO-VID-19 vaccination as it resumes recreational cruises in 2021 and beyond.

In the pre-pandemic era, the number of people who take to the seas for either short or long voyages is astonishingly high. It's estimated that 30 million passengers are transported annually on 272 ships worldwide.

Shortly after SARS-CoV-2 emerged, these vessels garnered a reputation as floating incubators of coronavirus infection for the same reason that anyplace where people congregate in large numbers can become sites of SARS-CoV-2 spread. The ships have hundreds, sometimes thousands of people on board, a population that includes passengers and crew members. There are parties, dances, and restaurant- and buffet-style dining. There are fitness classes and shows featuring entertainers. All of these activities bring passengers into close proximity with each other. In terms of time, a cruise can last for as few as two to five days or as long as 14 weeks for voyages around the globe. The shared spaces and ventilation systems can promote superspreader events.

In a CDC study of coronavirus outbreaks aboard major luxury liners, the agency found more than 800 cases of laboratory-confirmed COVID-19 were linked to outbreaks on three cruise ships in early 2020. These outbreaks also were associated with multiple deaths. The ship with the most COVID-19 morbidity and mortality was *Diamond Princess,* which left Yokohama, Japan, on January 20, 2020, with 3,700 passengers and crew members on board. More than 700 COVID-19 cases were associated with the ship; 567 passengers ultimately tested positive, as did 145 crew members. Most of the deaths were among older travelers. Indeed, the first two deaths, which were recorded on February 19, were an 87-year-old man and an 84-year-old woman. One 80-year-old passenger who had disembarked in Hong Kong, before it was known that COVID-19 was spreading on board, later tested positive as well. The Hong Kong resident's positive test is a reminder that passengers who disembark can unwittingly spread the virus to family and friends not associated with the voyage.

PART SIX

Viruses 101: Superspreaders, Long Haulers, and Testing

What is a virus?

What are the key features of a pandemic virus?

What is an RNA virus?

More . . .

58. What is a virus?

Virus

A submicroscopic infectious agent that requires living cells of a host to replicate and survive.

Viruses are some of the smallest infectious entities known to biology, and they are *the* most common type of pathogen that afflicts humans. Perhaps one of the most difficult things to wrap your head around when it comes to viruses, aside from their colossal power to cause mass casualties, is their infinitesimal, submicroscopic size. Viruses are inconceivably tiny. The only other infectious agents that are comparatively as small are the rogue proteins known as prions, which are linked to degenerative brain diseases, such as kuru and Creutzfeldt-Jakob disease. Prions measure about 100 nanometers in size. But the tiniest viruses—members of the Parvoviridae and Picornaviridae families—are even smaller, measuring about 20 to 30 nanometers in diameter. A nanometer is barely imaginable—one-billionth of a meter.

SARS-CoV-2 is hefty by comparison, measuring about 120 nanometers, although it's sometimes smaller. But SARS-CoV-2 comes nowhere near the largest viruses in sheer size, distinctions that belong to members of the Mimiviridae and Poxviridae families. Mimiviruses, which invade algae, are whoppers at 750 nanometers. Poxviruses, although large (about 400 nanometers), are noteworthy for more than just their size: The variola virus, a member of this family, is the cause of the disfiguring and deadly smallpox disease, which killed more than 300 million people in the 20th century alone.

The death toll from smallpox is a prime example of what happens when a highly transmissible virus continues moving through susceptible human populations. Herd immunity doesn't occur; infection and death do. Smallpox, an invisible enemy, plagued global populations from 600 A.D. until 1977, when the last case of natural infection occurred. There was one case of laboratory infection the following year, but in 1980, smallpox became the only infectious disease ever declared eradicated. An aggressive vaccination campaign led to the elimination of smallpox from human circulation. The only remaining stocks of the virus are in vials at high-containment laboratories in two countries—the United States and Russia. The U.S. vials are maintained under exceptionally tight security at the CDC. The Russian vials are at the State Research Center of Virology and Biotechnology (VECTOR Institute) in Koltsovo, Russia. These remaining smallpox stocks are maintained under the supervision of the WHO.

Even though poxviruses and miniviruses are large enough to be visible with a light microscope, they are still super small, and a reminder that tiny entities can have titanic consequences. SARS-CoV-2 is minuscule but it spawned a pandemic that swept rapidly around the world: tiny virus, gargantuan consequences. That's the same juxtaposition between SARS-CoV-2 and the pandemic that has swept around the world: tiny virus, gargantuan consequences. Molecular biologist, Dr. Arthur Levine, discoverer of the tumor suppressor gene, p53, has written prolifically about constituents of the microscopic and submicroscopic world that are difficult to imagine because of their infinitesimal size. Levine wrote in his classic text, *Viruses*, that for centuries people have been fascinated by the concepts of largest and smallest. For mathematicians, the notions of largest and smallest are best understood in the comparison between infinity and zero. For physicists, Levine defined the juxtaposition as the vastness of an ever-expanding universe opposite the imponderable smallness of particles smaller than atoms. Among biologists, Levine mused, there's respect for the grandeur of whales and redwood trees and equal respect for the awesome power of the entities at the opposite end of the size spectrum: viruses. They are unique in nature for a variety of reasons—not just their infinitesimal size or the sometimes deadly power they hold over their hosts, triggering outbreaks, epidemics, and pandemics.

Obligate parasite

An organism or other entity, such as a virus, that is entirely dependent on the living cells of its host.

Viruses are the ultimate freeloaders, defined more judiciously by virologists as **obligate parasites**, which means they are entirely dependent on the living cells of their hosts to survive regardless of whether the host is a plant, an animal, or a human. Viruses do not respire, move independently, or grow, and they lack metabolic processes. Yet they are the most abundant "life-form" on the planet, even though some scientists contend that viruses fail to meet the basic definition of life because of obligate parasitism. Still, they remain the most common cause of infections.

Countless viruses are harbored by animals in the wild. Over the past several decades many have increasingly jumped the species barrier to infect humans. Most instances can be blamed on human encroachment into ancient habitats. Betacoronaviruses, the general category to which the three lethal coronaviruses belong, are naturally harbored by bats. Two coronaviruses that cause the common cold (OC43 and HKU1) are also betacoronaviruses. But bats, as it turns out, are the ancient reservoir of alpha coronaviruses, the category to which the coronaviruses, 229E and NL63 belong. Both also cause the common cold. Clearly, bat-linked pathogens have been an long-time source of human infection.

Although viruses can trigger extremely complex diseases, such as AIDS, Ebola, rabies, yellow fever, and some forms of cancer, there really isn't much to these infectious agents. They're relatively simple structures. All have a set of genes (RNA or DNA), which are encased in a **capsid**, a protein shell that protects the genetic material inside. Some, like SARS-CoV-2 and its cousin coronaviruses, are known as **enveloped viruses**, which means they also have a greasy overcoat that swaths the capsid. The entire individual entity, comprised of genes, capsid, and fatty overcoat is known as a **virion**.

In addition to coronaviruses, influenza, Ebola, and hepatitis B and C viruses are on a formidable list of enveloped viruses. These viruses obtain their fatty coats from host cell membranes through a process called **budding**. Host cell structures have a double lipid layer and as the virus "buds off" in search of other cells to infect, it becomes enveloped in fat, taking a piece of you with it! This fat is quite vulnerable to soap, which is why handwashing is so important. Soap is like kryptonite to enveloped viruses.

59. What are the key features of a pandemic virus?

In *Global Catastrophic Biological Risks*, a book published about a month before the COVID-19 pandemic erupted, Drs. Thomas V. Inglesby and Amesh Adalja explained in intricate detail Nature's recipe for a pandemic virus, which differs from viral infectious agents that cause limited or seasonal infections. The book outlines traits shared by pandemic viruses regardless of the viral family from which they emerge. Both scientists are experts in infectious diseases at the Johns Hopkins University Bloomberg School of Public Health's Center for Health Security.

When a pathogen has the capacity to cause a pandemic, it will possess several attributes that aren't evident among

Capsid
A protein shell that protects the genetic material inside a virus.

Enveloped viruses
Viruses that have a fatty overcoat that surrounds the capsid.

Virion
The entire microbial entity composed of genes, capsid, and, if present, fatty overcoat.

Budding
The process by which a virion replicates itself and emerges from a cell to seek out and infect other cells.

seasonally circulating infectious agents. The most devastating pandemic viruses meet several key criteria:

1. The virus is spread via respiratory transmission;
2. The virus is capable of spreading during the incubation period prior to symptom onset;
3. Hosts have no preexisting immunity to the viral agent.

Those criteria leap from the page of the Inglesby and Adalja book, a slim volume of 135 pages, because they so accurately describe SARS-CoV-2, the virus that spawned the global COVID-19 pandemic. Stunningly, the book was published in November of 2019, a month before the outbreak was reported in Wuhan, China.

Virus trackers have known for years that a novel respiratory pathogen poses the greatest danger for pandemic spread, but Inglesby and Adalja recognized as their second criterion that transmission can occur during the incubation period before symptoms emerge. In effect, they predicted presymptomatic and asymptomatic transmission of SARS-CoV-2. By way of comparison, studies have shown that seasonal flu can be spread by asymptomatic carriers, but not at the same transmission rate of symptomatic individuals.

Both asymptomatic and presymptomatic transmission of SARS-CoV-2 were openly debated in the early months of the pandemic. Many doubters, who frequently based their reasoning in politics, not science, thought it was impossible for SARS-CoV-2 to be transmitted among people without symptoms.

As for respiratory transmission in general, any infection that spreads by way of droplets and aerosols can result in rapid transmission because the pathogen can be widely broadcast in confined spaces, such as classrooms, offices, bars, restaurants, or movie theaters—basically anywhere people congregate. And public health officials have seen non-pandemic respiratory viruses proliferate for the same reasons. "The prolific spread of influenza, pertussis, measles, and rhinoviruses is testament to this fact," Inglesby and Adalja wrote.

Controlling a pandemic driven by respiratory droplets and aerosols therefore becomes more difficult without the benefit of a vaccine. This aerial mode of transmission not only promotes prolific viral spread, it also underlies rapid increases in the hospitalization of critically ill patients—those suffering from pneumonia or acute respiratory distress syndrome (ARDS), necessitating the need for a ventilator.

Among the many concerns throughout major surges in pandemic cases was whether there would be enough ventilators for patients in need. During a devastating summer peak in Texas cases, hospitals turned away transfer patients because beds and ventilators were in low supply. Stopping the spread of SARS-CoV-2 became difficult throughout the Sunbelt for weeks as governments refused to mandate face masks and physical distancing measures. A key fact that never quite struck home with people who politicized the pandemic is that an incalculable number of virus particles are released by infected individuals as they talk, or when they cough or sneeze. "Interventions to interrupt [respiratory] spread are more difficult to implement when the simple and universal act of breathing can spread a pathogen," Inglesby and Adalja asserted. In contrast, they noted that even though some pathogens spread prolifically via the fecal-oral route, such as *Vibrio cholerae* and the hepatitis A virus—both of which generate explosive epidemics—"a modicum of sanitary infrastructure can quench the outbreak."

60. What is an RNA virus?

The hereditary information in all coronaviruses is stored in the genetic material known as **ribonucleic acid (RNA)**, a critical macromolecule vital to life on Earth. **Deoxyribonucleic acid (DNA)** is the form in which higher forms of life—everything from humans to bumblebees to banana trees, birds, snakes, sharks, fungi, bacteria, algae, and a whole lot more—package their genetic information. For humans, DNA is the double-stranded master molecule of life that contains the genetic code. Although SARS-CoV-2 stores its genetic material in RNA, other viruses package their genetic information in either RNA or DNA. Complex forms of life have both DNA and RNA. Humans, for example, have multiple forms of RNA, such as messenger RNA, ribosomal RNA, and transfer RNA. The primary role of RNA in higher organisms is to convert the information stored in DNA into proteins.

When it comes to the genetics of viruses, these infectious agents abide by a unique set of rules, all of which aid and abet their parasitism—and survival. Viral genes carry instructions to help the pathogen elude the human immune system or pick the perfect lock on the surface of cells that will allow them to slip inside. Although a virus can store its genes in either RNA or DNA, no virus possesses both. The genes can be strung along a single strand, or they can be double strands of either RNA or DNA.

Coronaviridae is a family of **single-stranded RNA viruses**, but it isn't the only viral family whose members

Ribonucleic acid (RNA)

The spiraling master molecule of life that contains the genetic code for all higher forms of life. This includes animals, plants, bacteria, archaea, and protists. DNA is in each cell and determines when and which life-sustaining proteins to make.

Deoxyribonucleic acid (DNA)

The macromolecule that contains the genetic code.

Single-stranded RNA viruses

Viruses such as SARS-CoV-2 that encode their genetic information in a single strand of RNA.

store their genetic material in RNA. Those that do so form a large and diverse group of highly infectious viruses, many potentially lethal. Some of these viruses include those that cause influenza, dengue, Ebola disease, measles, polio, rabies, and West Nile fever. These viruses are in no way similar just because they are single-stranded RNA viruses. SARS-CoV-2, for example, has a genome that is more than twice the size of the influenza virus genome.

Numerous other differences separate one viral family from another. Each virus family is endowed with genes that dictate wildly different instructions aimed at that specific infectious agent's survival. You may recall from earlier in the discussion (Question 58) that some viruses, like SARS-CoV-2, are enveloped, but other RNA viruses, such as poliovirus, are non-enveloped. And there are subtler and more complex differences among viral families, factors that allow virologists to categorize these pathogens in minute molecular detail.

All of this provides some grounding in the incredible diversity among viruses and the diverse diseases they cause. The list of RNA viruses doesn't end with the few outlined so far in this text. There is not only a long list of additional single-stranded RNA viruses but an equally long list of other features that virologists rely on to classify them.

Yet, just as there are single-stranded RNA viruses, there are viruses whose genes are stored in two strands of RNA, a class of viruses known as double-stranded RNA viruses. This category of viruses includes rotavirus, which causes intestinal infections, and Colorado tick fever virus, transmitted by Rocky Mountain wood ticks. This rare but mild infection has been periodically detected in the western United States and as far north as Canada.

On the whole, whether single or double stranded, RNA viruses have high mutation rates in common. This high mutation rate results in several slightly different versions of the viral genome being made each time the genome is replicated, according to scientists at the Johns Hopkins Center for Health Security.

SARS-CoV-2's genome produces proteins that aid its ability to break and enter into human cells, hijack cell processes, and replicate itself. In terms of the genetic alphabet—the entire genome of SARS-CoV-2 is approximately 30,000 "letters" in length. The letters are derived from the alphabet: AUCG, which stands for the chemicals adenine, uracil, cytosine, and guanine. From this alphabet, various combinations of those letters spell out the code for 10 genes that produce 29 proteins. By comparison, influenza A viruses have eight genes that are derived from 13,500 letters of the same genetic alphabet, AUCG. Those letters also spell out the code for proteins that drive SARS-CoV-2's ability to escape immune system forces.

At first glance, it may seem confusing that 10 genes can produce more than 20 proteins. But apparently one gene carries the code for a so-called polyprotein. The whopper protein is snipped into more than 15 proteins by molecular scissors that SARS-CoV-2 packs in its genetic tool kit.

By comparison, humans have a genetic alphabet also comprised of only four letters: ATCG (T is for thymine), a genome of 3 billion letters to spell out the 30,000 genes in the human genome. For the record, humans have multiple forms of RNA. You've likely heard of messenger RNA (mRNA), endowed with the crucial role of copying sequences of DNA, which carry the codes for proteins required by the cell. There are other critical forms of RNA, such as ribosomal RNA and transfer RNA, but it's important to make a mental note of mRNA because it will be addressed again in the discussion about vaccines.

61. How did viruses evolve?

There are three theories on viral evolution—where viruses came from in the first place. We know that many are carried by animals, particularly bats, such as the horseshoe bat, which is believed to have been the animal that harbored the precursor virus that became SARS-CoV, the virus that caused the devastating SARS outbreak in the early 2000s. But some scientists have dug deeper and looked farther in an attempt to tease out how viruses not only became the most pervasive causes of infectious diseases, but why they've persisted for countless millennia on Earth and are the most abundant life-form on the planet.

Here are three prominent hypotheses examining how viruses came to be:

1. **Viruses Emerged First Hypothesis** is a notion that suggests viruses, possibly RNA viruses, existed before complex entities, such as cells.

2. **The Escape Hypothesis** posits that viruses arose from mobile snippets of genetic material that gained the ability to escape from one type of primordial cell only to invade another—and another and another. Each mobile snippet—virus—dependent on each cell for its very survival. In this hypothesis, cells came first. This is also known as the **Progressive Hypothesis**.

3. The **Regressive Hypothesis** argues that viruses may have evolved from free-living ancestors.

Dr. David Wessner of Davidson College, writing in *Nature Education*, noted that "existing viruses may have evolved from more complex, possibly free-living organisms that lost genetic information over time, as they adopted a parasitic approach to replication." He cites as possible examples large viruses such as Poxviridae and the enormous Mimiviridae (750 nanometers) as having evolved from free-living ancestors.

62. What does mutation mean, and do mutations mean that SARS-CoV-2 is likely to get worse?

Mutation

Changes that occur in genetic information.

Mutation sounds like a scary word, but it simply means changes to the genetic code—and viruses, especially RNA viruses, consistently mutate. SARS-CoV-2 is no exception. Mutations cause alterations in the sequence of AUGC molecules that make up SARS-CoV-2's genome.

Changes in the sequence of AUGC in SARS-CoV-2's genome were noted just months into the pandemic, when scientists around the world had already detected more than a dozen mutations in SARS-CoV-2's spike protein, also referred to as the "S" protein.

The virus uses its spikes to bind to the ACE2 receptor on human cells to initiate infection. The mutations were largely in the viral region known as the receptor binding domain (RBD). Mutations in the RBD have aided SARS-CoV-2's ability to fuse with cells it's trying to invade. SARS-CoV-2 also has other proteins that are more stable and do not mutate rapidly at all. Their stability is important to the overall function of the virus.

Scientists at the Johns Hopkins Center for Health Security have underscored that "RNA viruses have high mutation rates that result in several slightly different versions of the viral genome being made each time the viral genome is replicated. This creates a viral population with diverse genomes, known as quasispecies. With each viral replication cycle, the differences accumulate between the original viral genome and the progeny viral genomes."

Kai Kupferschmidt of *Science* magazine wrote: "On average, the coronavirus accumulates about two changes per month in its genome," which are common across the vast majority of SARS-CoV-2 variants in circulation globally. Staying abreast of these changes "helps researchers follow how the virus spreads. Most of the changes don't affect how the virus behaves, but a few may change the disease's transmissibility or severity," Kupferschmidt emphasized.

Dr. Bjorn Meyer, who studies RNA viruses at the Pasteur Institute in Paris, said in an interview for this book that viral mutation is not invariably geared toward extremes. In fact, evolution steers viruses toward survival—and SARS-CoV-2 won't survive if it's so lethal the majority of hosts die, Meyer contends.

"The most important feature for any virus is to be transmitted to its next host," Meyer explained. "This holds true for viruses that infect animals, plants, or humans. If a virus causes the death of its host, that means the virus can no longer transmit—and that becomes a dead end."

Examples from recent and past history illustrate how pandemic viruses change to ensure their survival. The 2009 pandemic H1N1 flu now circulates as a seasonal influenza virus, as does the pandemic virus that caused the explosive 1918 pandemic. It's still circulating episodically, causing sniffles, aches, and seasonal misery.

"If the host stays alive longer, then the virus can spread to additional hosts for a longer period of time," Meyer asserted. "This often means that viruses that cause high mortality rates are often [weeded out] in the longer process of viral evolution and we're left with more adapted, less virulent viruses."

Meyer further noted that since SARS-CoV-2 only recently spilled over from an animal reservoir into humans, it is not well adapted to the human environment. "Under certain circumstances, one could compare it to a bull in a china shop. During the course of infection, it triggers certain pathways and immune responses that cause COVID-19 to be fatal for some people. Over a long period of time one would expect it to become less lethal, but this might require many years of evolution."

The B.1.1.7 variant of SARS-CoV-2 that emerged in Britain in November of 2020, quickly spread around the world. The mutations that made the variant successful occurred in the spike protein, which the virus uses to attach to host cells. The variant is more contagious because it is better adapted to infiltrate. That feature doesn't make it more lethal.

63. Where in the body does SARS-CoV-2 proliferate most?

As mentioned earlier, SARS-CoV-2 is a respiratory virus, spread primarily through droplets and aerosols. The pathogen has an affinity for the upper respiratory tract. Viral proliferation in this region explains why acquiring a sample for laboratory testing involves nasal and throat swabbing. Cells in the nasal passages and throat have an abundance of ACE2 receptors, the preferred passageway into cells by SARS-CoV-2. This is why the virus is so easily transmitted through the innocuous acts of breathing, talking, coughing, and sneezing. That said, there are other medical problems that arise as a direct consequence of infection (Question 66). Researchers have found that severe COVID-19 can be characterized by excessive blood clotting, kidney impairment, and strokes. A growing number of people have reported struggling with post-COVID conditions, such as extraordinary fatigue, headaches, and a disparate range of other medical conditions (Question 66). Even though the infection may begin in the respiratory tract and can develop into acute respiratory distress syndrome for some patients, it can morph in the post-COVID-19 period into chronic conditions that last for weeks to months.

Dr. Bjorn Meyer of the Pasteur Institute in Paris explained that SARS-CoV-2 differs from its cousin coronaviruses, SARS-CoV and MERS-CoV, in the respiratory tract sites that it preferentially attacks. "The other viruses seem to primarily infect the lower respiratory tract," Meyer said of the agents that cause SARS and MERS, "therefore it might be slightly more difficult for them to spread between humans. SARS-CoV-2, however, seems to replicate well in the upper respiratory tract, grows there quickly to high viral loads, and is able to transmit between humans, who spread it simply by droplets produced during breathing and coughing, quite well. Taking this into consideration, it may seem less surprising that this virus spreads so well and has spread around the world in such a short period of time, especially in this tightly connected society we are living in."

This shouldn't be construed as representing the only sites where the virus infects its hosts. Like its counterparts, SARS-CoV and MERS-CoV, the pandemic coronavirus infects the lungs. But SARS-CoV-2 also infects the gastrointestinal tract, the eyes, middle ear, and the kidneys. The virus so profoundly attacks the senses of smell and taste that Dr. Rachel Batterham of University College London says the loss of smell (anosmia) and taste should be recognized as COVID-19 symptoms.

In a study published in the Public Library of Science Medicine (*PLoS Medicine*), Batterham and her colleagues found in a study of 567 participants with smell and taste loss that 78% had SARS-CoV-2 antibodies. Indeed, those whose sense of smell apparently had been robbed by the infection were three times more likely to have the antibodies than those who lost sense of taste alone. This suggested to Batterham and her team that loss of smell is highly specific to COVID-19.

64. Are superspreaders and superspreader events real?

Superspreaders

Individuals who disproportionately transmit an infection to multiple people.

Superspreader events

A documentable single event that promotes the spread of an infectious disease to large numbers of people.

20/80 rule

A general rule in infectious disease transmission that 1 in 5 people spreads infections within a population and controls most transmission events.

Both **superspreaders** and **superspreader events** are genuine and have been documented in other infectious diseases, but it took the COVID-19 pandemic to rivet an international spotlight on the phenomenon. Studies as far back as 1997 have defined and used the terms *superspreader* and *superspreader events*. Asymptomatic and presymptomatic transmission apparently are key factors in superspreading events. But the phenomenon has been described in the medical literature for more than a century, long before the term superspreader came into vogue.

Public health scientists have long emphasized the **20/80 rule** of infectious disease transmission. That is, approximately 1 in 5 people spreads infections within any population, and this proportion of transmitters has been observed to control most transmission events. This empirical rule is the foundation for superspreaders, and it has been shown to hold sway over the transmission dynamics for many pathogens in multiple species. Some individuals disproportionately infect more secondary contacts than the majority in any given population.

In the case of SARS-CoV-2, the virus concentrates in the nasopharynx region, which is conducive to spreading the virus through the simple acts of breathing, speaking, coughing, etc. Dr. Bjorn Meyer (Question 63) explains SARS-CoV-2 establishes itself and replicates quickly in the upper respiratory tract, reaching high viral loads. One of the key reasons for face mask recommendations is blunting the passage of an easily transmittable virus.

Examples of SARS-CoV-2 superspreading events have been extraordinary. Health officials in South Korea reported the case of "Patient 31," a prolific superspreader and member of the fringe church called Shincheonji. Patient 31 is believed to have been the source of about 5,000 SARS-CoV-2 infections.

Anecdotal reports of coronavirus-associated super-spreader events abound worldwide. In the state of Washington, 61 members of a choir in Skagit County met for their weekly rehearsal in March 2020. One person at the choir practice, which ran approximately 2½ hours, displayed cold-like symptoms, according to the CDC. Within days, 53 COVID-19 cases were identified by the agency (87% of the singers), and two members of the group later died as a direct consequence of the infection. Singing forces more viruses from the respiratory tract into the surrounding environment, scientists have found.

In Millinocket, Maine, a wedding on August 8, 2020, was the event that led to 30 infections among attendees.

But 140 additional people who didn't go to the wedding were infected as a result of secondary transmission, eight of those people died of COVID-19. None of the wedding attendees died. However, the effects of the single superspreader event didn't end there.

A fairly significant number of people in the secondary outbreak (74 cases) were infected because one attendee worked at a jail, 240 miles away from the initial event. Public health investigators who analyzed the event concluded that the explosive number of cases illustrates how quickly chains of transmission evolve.

No superspreader event was more surprising than the one that occurred at the White House during a Rose Garden ceremony in September 2020. The event, which was organized to introduce Donald Trump's Supreme Court nominee, resulted in at least 35 direct infections, which included Trump, his wife Melania, many senior White House staffers, several senators, and former New Jersey Governor Chris Christie, who wound up in an intensive care unit for several days. No single source was ever identified as the cause of the infections.

The White House event was a stunning example of what *not* to do during a pandemic. From the pandemic's start, Trump openly flouted mask-wearing and public health recommendations, a model mimicked by his followers and members of his political party. This event showed why this behavior is a recipe for disaster. Although the ceremony was held outdoors, the crowd was large and densely packed. There was no social distancing, hardly any mask wearers, and it was an extraordinarily bad example for a country, which at that time had already experienced more than 200,000 deaths. Videos of the event revealed hugging, handshaking, and close face-to-face conversations.

Just for the record, superspreaders and superspreading events have been documented throughout relatively recent and distant history involving other infectious diseases. During the SARS pandemic in 2003, a 54-year-old-man admitted to a hospital in China for diabetes and kidney failure wound up infecting 33 people in the hospital. The patient had not been diagnosed with the infection; however, he was in contact with someone who had an active case. The man died of SARS. He has been dubbed a superspreader, and the hospital outbreak was thus a superspreader event. In 1989, a measles outbreak in rural Finland has been defined as a classic superspreader event with one notable superspreader. The outbreak occurred in a school, where 51 cases were counted by health officials. However, one child was found to have infected 22 people. Deeper in history, Mary Mallon ("Typhoid Mary"), a New York domestic worker who in the early 20th century was identified as a carrier of *Salmonella typhi*, the bacterial infection that causes typhoid fever, has been declared a noteworthy superspreader. She was said to have infected at least 51 people, and possibly many more, over a period of about 15 years.

65. Will SARS-CoV-2 become endemic?

The CDC refers to an **endemic disease** as one that has a constant presence and/or usual prevalence in a population. **Hyperendemic disease** refers to a disease that occurs at persistently high levels in a population. The SARS-CoV-2 virus is so new to the global community that medical and scientific experts have yet to determine with any degree of certainty whether SARS-CoV-2 will become endemic.

Endemic disease

A disease that has a constant or typical prevalence in a community.

Hyperendemic disease

A disease that has a high prevalence within a community or population.

Widespread vaccinations can help mitigate SARS-CoV-2 infections. Scientists at NIAID have predicted herd immunity is possible if 80% of people in the United States are vaccinated. Nevertheless, Hans Heesterbeek, in an essay in the online publication, *The Conversation*, argues that it's possible SARS-CoV-2 "will eventually stabilize at a constant level so that it becomes present in communities at all times, possibly at a relatively low, sometimes predictable rate. This is what we mean when we say a disease is endemic," he said.

Heesterbeek, a professor of theoretical epidemiology at Utrecht University in the Netherlands, further noted that when there is consistent spread in a geographic area (which can refer to an entire country or several countries), endemic transmission becomes a genuine possibility. "Theoretically speaking, an infection becomes endemic if, on average, each infected individual transmits it to one person. In other words, when the reproduction number $(R) = 1$. In comparison, during an epidemic when the spread of the disease is increasing, R is more than 1, and when the spread is decreasing through control measures (vaccination, for example) or population immunity, R is less than 1."

66. What is "long COVID"? Does the virus linger for months?

Long COVID refers to symptoms that emerge after the virus has waned, which become persistent and often debilitating lasting weeks to months. Many of these patients call themselves "long haulers."

Symptoms of long COVID run a wide and disparate gamut: headaches, crushing fatigue, dizziness, tachycardia, shortness of breath, prediabetes, high blood pressure, and fevers, to name a few.

"Anecdotally, there's no question that there are a considerable number of individuals who have a post-viral syndrome that really, in many respects, can incapacitate them for weeks and weeks following so-called recovery and clearing of the virus," Dr. Anthony Fauci, director of the National Institute of Allergy and Infectious Diseases said during a webinar on COVID-19 in July 2020. Fauci and other experts in infectious diseases say it will take in-depth studies to uncover the full scope of the pandemic coronavirus's aftereffects and how long they last.

Some people who've weathered the infection think they're already well aware of the sweeping range of symptoms that can linger long after the virus has cleared. Diana Berrent, a COVID-19 survivor in Port Washington, New York, founded an organization called Survivor Corps and says 98 distinct persisting medical problems can occur as a direct consequence of having had COVID-19. "Some people are experiencing tremendous neurological issues—aphasia and strokes," said Berrent, who describes herself as having been a "Tylenol and Gatorade" COVID patient—meaning, one who responded to COVID-19 by self-quarantining at home and treating herself with over-the-counter remedies. She was not hospitalized.

Berrent oversees a Facebook group of 110,000 COVID-19 long haulers, a centerpiece of her Survivor Corps. She describes the group as unique mainly because it's the only one of COVID long haulers, who self-isolated at home as she did. Although Berrent estimates that 1 in 3 people experiences lingering aftereffects following a COVID-19 diagnosis, a British study of post-COVID patients put the number at 1 in 20.

For some people, post-COVID symptoms last for a few weeks. Others, like Berrent, have ongoing health problems months after COVID-19. "I felt like my brain was about to pop out of my skull," she said of her own bouts with neurological problems. Members of her organization, which in addition to the Facebook presence has a website, are reporting serious medical issues. "People are starting to report dental issues and a lot of ocular issues. One of the big ones is a lot of GI issues. We have young people in our group who are in wheelchairs. It's almost as if they have aged decades in only a few months," Berrent said.

She said her group of 110,000 post-COVID survivors has become a goldmine of information for medical scientists seeking to understand long COVID. Survivors have participated in surveys and have conveyed to doctors what it's like when the aftereffects of COVID-19 can't be shaken off. "Many people have spoken of feeling as if they're in a fog," said Berrent, who added that most long haulers are women.

"People are in pain, genuine pain. Some say they have a feeling of electrical bolts coursing through their bodies. Others have extreme hair loss. You name it—COVID toes have been a problem," she said of a rash that appears on the toes of some people.

"I have had terrible deep ear pain," said Berrent, who added that glaucoma has developed in one eye, which she said is part of her constellation of problems that have grown out of a bout with COVID-19. She and members of her organization aren't alone among people who have faced difficult recoveries.

New York Times editorial writer Mara Gay, who has appeared frequently on cable television news broadcasts, has spoken openly about her bout with COVID-19, which left her feeling "not herself" for months afterward. Gay, who described herself as an avid runner prior to her diagnosis, said it took months before she could run the same distances and at the same pace. At the height of her illness, she described her lungs as feeling as if they were filled with tar.

67. Is SARS-CoV-2 reinfection possible?

Case reports have begun to emerge that suggest reinfection is possible after having successfully cleared the coronavirus from an earlier infection. The first U.S. case study was reported in the journal *Lancet Infectious Diseases* by medical scientists from the University of Nevada, Reno School of Medicine and the Nevada State Public Health Laboratory. The case involved a 25-year-old Nevada man who presented to health authorities on two occasions with symptoms of viral infection. He was symptomatic in March 2020, tested positive for SARS-CoV-2 at a community testing event in April, 2020, then (after symptoms resolved) tested negative in two follow-up tests in May before becoming symptomatic once more at the end of that month. He received positive tests when he went to a primary care clinician and subsequently to a hospital in early June. The team of medical scientists who reported the case said nasopharyngeal swabs were obtained at each visit and twice during follow-up. Positive tests were obtained each time he was symptomatic—but what makes this case interesting is that two *different* variants of SARS-CoV-2 were identified from swabs taken on different occasions.

The findings suggest the patient was infected by SARS-CoV-2 on two separate occasions by genetically distinct SARS-CoV-2 variants. The team concluded that "previous exposure to SARS-CoV-2 might not guarantee total immunity in all cases." Having isolated genetically distinct viruses also suggested to the Nevada medical investigators the patient was not suffering a relapse. At the time of the report, the case was the fifth reinfection episode reported worldwide. The others were reported in Ecuador, Hong Kong, the Netherlands, and Belgium.

In guidance posted on its website, the CDC has taken a more cautious stance, emphasizing that it is impossible to say whether someone can be reinfected. "Data to date show that [anyone] who has had and recovered from COVID-19 may have low levels of virus in their bodies for up to 3 months after diagnosis," agency officials wrote. "This means that if the person who has recovered from COVID-19 is retested within three months of initial infection, they may continue to have a positive test result."

But the Nevada team made certain their tests did not involve the same virus by running a polymerase chain reaction (PCR) test (Question 72) on each of the patient's test samples. PCR testing revealed viruses with substantially different genetic signatures, findings that confirmed to the team their patient had been infected on separate occasions.

Contact tracing
The process of identifying and contacting persons who have been in close contact with a person confirmed to have an infectious disease.

68. What is contact tracing, and does it help lower rates of infection?

The goal of **contact tracing** is to alert as many people as possible who may have been exposed to someone with a confirmed coronavirus infection. The basic rule for contact tracing is to identify **"close contacts,"** which are defined as persons who have been within 6 feet of an infected person for at least 10 minutes. Such close contacts would be urged to isolate themselves and monitor for symptoms. The goal is to break potential new chains of transmission; thus, if one of the contacts is found to be symptomatic, that person would be asked for the identities of close contacts so that the contact tracing would begin anew. There are apps that have been developed for cell phones that make contact tracing easier. The drawback to contact tracing is that tracers' phone calls frequently go unreturned, and in instances of a large outbreak or surge, the effort may be futile.

Whether contact tracing is effective in preventing disease transmission is still unclear. In concept, particularly with a disease that "hides" the way asymptomatic COVID-19 does, alerting people to potential exposure may be the only way to keep them from spreading it to others. In practice, though, contact tracing is a tough job: Delays can be caused by the infected person's lack of symptoms. It may be difficult reaching close contacts, or contacts may have trouble accessing testing to confirm infections. These problems—and many others—can reduce the effectiveness of contact tracing as a way of preventing disease spread.

69. How do I know if I have been exposed to SARS-CoV-2?

There are several types of tests that can be performed to determine whether exposure has occurred in the recent past, or if you are currently infected with the virus. Your healthcare provider will determine which type of test is best for you based on your personal history and whether you currently have symptoms.

Close contact
A person who has been within 6 feet or less of an infected individual for more than 10 minutes.

Among the most searing photos that define the COVID-19 pandemic—the largest in more than a century—show people standing in lines or waiting in cars (sometimes for miles) to have nasal or throat swabs performed by a healthcare provider. It's important to understand that the swab itself isn't a test per se. The swabs provide a **specimen** that can produce a result using any one of several forms of **diagnostic testing**. Saliva specimens also are used for specialized testing. The home-based SARS-CoV-2 detection test by Quest Diagnostics is a nasal swab test, which is sent to you and returned to the company by overnight mail. Other types of tests will be discussed in Questions 70–72.

70. What is an antibody test?

An **antibody test** determines if there has been a past infection of SARS-CoV-2. This kind of test is a blood test (also known as a **serology** test) that is designed to detect antibodies, the proteins produced by plasma cells (B lymphocytes) of the immune system.

Antibody tests generally are ordered when you've had symptoms that you felt may have been mild COVID-19, but you recovered. Or, you were exposed to someone who was diagnosed with the infection. Your immune system produces several different kinds of antibodies. Testing is available to detect two types of these proteins:

1. **Binding antibodies**. These are antibodies that latch onto the virus. Even though you may have a positive test for binding antibodies, the results cannot give your clinician information on how extensively you may have been infected.

2. An evolving type of test can detect **neutralizing antibodies**. This test is performed after a positive test for binding antibodies.

Specimen

Tissue or fluids collected for examination and diagnostic testing.

Diagnostic testing

Any of several types of tests that can identify the presence of disease.

Antibody test

A blood test that looks for antibodies to a specific pathogen.

Serology

Investigations that examine blood samples.

Binding antibodies

Antibodies that latch onto a pathogen.

Neutralizing antibodies

Antibodies that make a pathogen incapable of replicating and continuing the infection.

An antibody test can determine that you've previously been exposed; however, it cannot determine whether you're currently infected. A question that remains unanswered is how long antibodies detected by these tests might provide immunity, especially in the event of a new infection. Doctors as yet do not have enough evidence to say with certainty how long these antibodies remain viable or whether they guard against reinfection (see Question 67).

71. What is a rapid antigen test?

Rapid antigen tests can produce results within minutes and are designed to detect a current infection. Antigen tests pinpoint the presence of viral proteins—antigens. These tests are authorized by the U.S. Food and Drug Administration to be performed on nasopharyngeal or nasal swab specimens. Antigen tests are so-called point-of-care tests, which means they are performed at the site where the patient is seeking a result. By contrast, a PCR test (described in Question 72), which may take several days to return a result, is considered the gold standard among diagnostic tests for identifying SARS-CoV-2. This usually occurs in instances when a patient's specimen is sent to a laboratory offsite from the point of care. That said, the sensitivity of rapid antigen tests is generally lower than PCR, according to the CDC.

The CDC's guidance emphasizes that antigen levels in specimens collected beyond 5 to 7 days of the onset of symptoms may drop below the limit of detection of the test, resulting in a **false-negative test result**. A more sensitive test such as PCR, the CDC contends, will likely return a positive result.

Rapid antigen tests

Tests that identify viral proteins (antigens); they can produce results within minutes and are designed to detect a current infection.

False-negative test result

A test result that shows a patient to be negative for viral infection when in fact the patient is infected with the virus.

72. What is a PCR test, and how does it detect SARS-CoV-2?

Polymerase chain reaction (PCR)

A laboratory technique used routinely to identify sequences of DNA.

PCR stands for **polymerase chain reaction**, an indispensable laboratory technique that revolutionized the biological and medical sciences. PCR's inventor, the late Kary Banks Mullis, won the 1993 Nobel Prize in Chemistry for the innovation. In this answer we will first explore how PCR routinely functions in laboratories worldwide on non-viral samples then segue into an explanation of how it detects SARS-CoV-2.

PCR is used to make millions, even billions, of copies of DNA, a process called DNA amplification. The test can be conducted with just a single, often infinitesimal fragment of DNA. To name a few applications, the technology is used in the detection of tumor DNA; the identification of bacteria; aiding studies of DNA in biological research; police department forensics; and providing definitive answers in paternity testing. Scientists at the National Human Genome Research Institute refer to PCR as "molecular photocopying." The institute relied on PCR in its massive efforts to map the human genome. The technique is so powerful it has helped identify criminal suspects from trace amounts of DNA left in a single drop of blood at a crime scene.

PCR is very accurate, but it needs specialized equipment. It relies on a device called a thermocycler, in which the DNA sample is amplified exponentially—increased over 30 to 40 cycles of heating and cooling. During the process, DNA's two strands are pulled apart then recombined, increasing the amount of available DNA with each cycle. The amount of DNA is increased, providing a sequence that can be analyzed. After the first cycle, two separated strands of DNA (remember, DNA is a *double* helix) are multiplied to four strands. The process repeats with the four strands becoming eight, eight becoming 16, and so on.

But what does any of that have to do with detecting a virus? As was stated earlier in Question 60, SARS-CoV-2 is an RNA virus. As it turns out, PCR can be used with a high degree of precision to detect the presence of viral nucleic acid, RNA. The PCR test for SARS-CoV-2 is referred to as a reverse transcriptase polymerase chain reaction, or RT-PCR. Reverse transcriptase is an enzyme used in PCR to convert RNA into double-stranded DNA.

The RT-PCR test is conducted on a patient's sample obtained through a nasal or throat swab. When RNA transcriptase converts RNA into double-stranded DNA, the sample then goes by the name of complementary DNA, or cDNA. Just as the PCR process is operated through repeated cycles to amplify natural DNA, the thermocycler processes cDNA to target viral sequences.

There are other advantages to PCR testing. Some PCR tests can additionally produce an indication of a patient's viral load with a measure called the cycle threshold (CT). And, yet another PCR test, which goes by the name of Flu SC2 Multiplex Assay, can detect three viruses at the same time: SARS-CoV-2, influenza A, and influenza B. That enables the patient's doctor to learn whether a symptomatic patient has COVID-19 or influenza and treat him or her accordingly.

PART SEVEN

Vaccines, Therapeutics, and Convalescent Plasma

What is a vaccine?

How many COVID-19 vaccines exist?

Why were COVID-19 vaccine trials suspended?

More . . .

73. *What is a vaccine?*

Vaccine

Injection of a substance relative to a specific pathogen, triggering an immune response. Administered in a minuscule dose. The aim is to prevent future infections by that pathogen.

Vaccines rank among the most important medical interventions ever developed, "and they have saved more lives than anything in medicine, even more than antibiotics," explained Dr. Adhi Sharma, chief medical officer at Mount Sinai South Nassau in Oceanside, New York. A vaccine isn't a single type of intervention. Generally speaking, they can be created in a variety of ways. There are five basic types of vaccines:

1. Live attenuated vaccine (LAV), which is "weakened" in a laboratory. LAVs often prompt a strong immune response. The measles, mumps, and rubella combined vaccine as well as the rotavirus and intranasal flu vaccines are live attenuated preparations.

2. Inactivated vaccines use a "killed" pathogen. Examples: annual flu shot; inactivated polio and hepatitis A vaccines

3. Toxoid vaccines fight toxin-producing organisms, such as the tetanus bacterial-toxin.

4. Conjugate vaccines combine a weak "antigen with strong antigen." That means a weak protein or sugar structure that doesn't prompt a strong response is combined—conjugated—with a protein or that does. *Haemophilus influenzae* (Hib) is a conjugate vaccine.

5. Subunit vaccines include only a snippet instead of the entire pathogen. Also, that portion is produced through biochemical or recombinant DNA technologies. A widely administered subunit vaccine is the one for hepatitis B.

COVID-19 prompted a flurry of scientific creativity and has produced innovative forms of immunization, especially the two-dose shots based on RNA technology.

Sharma praised vaccines as the most important medical interventions of all time because of their stunning power to stop a disease before it starts and spreads through populations. Vaccines have been administered routinely in the United States for more than 200 years, starting with the smallpox inoculation. As a public health tool, vaccines have been instrumental in making a number of deadly diseases nonexistent to extremely rare: Smallpox was eradicated from circulation because of vaccination; measles, mumps, diphtheria, polio, and tetanus, among others, were largely driven into retreat. Many of these diseases, without vaccines, could have caused countless deaths and major disabilities, such as blindness, deafness, brain damage, or paralysis. The list of infectious diseases that have been controlled or made less worrisome because of vaccines is noteworthy: rotovirus, *Haemophilus influenzae B (HiB)*, influenza, pneumococcal pneumonia, chickenpox, and shingles, to name a few of the most common.

One of the most important points to understand about vaccines is that they do not function like medications—they don't "cure" a disease or help you recover from it. What makes vaccines unique is that they *prevent* infectious diseases from occurring in the first place.

The terms "vaccine" and "vaccination" are derived from the name of the cowpox virus—*vaccinia*—coined by English physician Edward Jenner, who developed the first widely used vaccine to prevent smallpox in 1796 (historical accounts suggest "vaccines" were in use long before the 18th century in China and Africa, but they didn't go by that name).

Both words, *vaccine* and *vaccination*, are derived from the Latin word *vacca*, which means cow. Jenner had noticed that milkmaids who were exposed to cowpox, an infection specific to cows, never developed smallpox, the leading cause of human death in the 18th century. He decided to use the crusted matter from sores of affected cows as a preventive to ward off smallpox. His serendipitous discovery not only worked, it paved the way for vaccines to be used as major public health tools. Vaccination campaigns based on his inoculation process were underway in Britain as well as the United States by the early 19th century.

Vaccines are based on a deceptively simple concept: If you prompt the immune system to recognize and take action against a pathogen before you encounter it, you won't get sick when faced with the infectious agent. The simplest way to do this is to "show" the pathogen to the immune system in very limited amounts. A vaccine can therefore "contain the same germs that cause the disease," reports the CDC, noting, for example, that "measles vaccine contains measles virus, and *Haemophilus influenzae* B vaccine contains HiB bacteria."

The theory behind vaccination as a public health tool is quite basic: People who are immunized against a communicable disease can avoid getting sick and passing the contagion on to others. No vaccine is 100% effective, but among those who are vaccinated, even if illness does occur, it's likely to be mild and far less encumbering than facing the infection without it. Unfortunately, vaccination doesn't intervene in a disease already in progress, so if you are already infected, getting vaccinated won't help. The COVID-19 pandemic helped change the concept of a vaccine and sparked a new era in the field of vaccinology. New types of vaccines have emerged because of the urgent need to gain the upper hand in an out-of-control pandemic. The United States had registered the highest number of cases and worst death rate on the entire planet, despite having many of the best scientists and public health experts in the world. A rampant anti-science stance that reached the highest levels of the U.S. government helped downplay the severity of the pandemic and left too many Americans unaware and unprepared.

The first COVID-19 vaccine in clinical trials was Moderna Therapeutics' messenger RNA (mRNA) vaccine (see Question 76), which immunized its first clinical trial volunteer in March 2020. Moderna, based in Cambridge, Massachusetts, was followed within 48 hours by China's CanSino Biologics announcing a clinical trial of its vaccine, which uses a deactivated adenovirus as a vehicle to deliver viral proteins into the individual being immunized. Many other vaccine candidates followed, some using similar technology to Moderna's and CanSino Biologics', others using different methods (see Question 75).

Regardless of how they are made, vaccines work by stimulating an immune response to the vaccine agent, which serves as a proxy for actual infection. The immune system creates neutralizing antibodies and a memory of the vaccine. This is exactly what happens in natural infection: The immune system detects the infectious agent and in so doing unleashes its potent forces, neutralizing it with antibodies and marking it for destruction via phagocytosis (see Question 44). A memory of the infiltrator is formed by the adaptive immune system (see Question 44), and the immune system is now primed to respond should the pathogen ever be encountered again. Despite vaccination simply exploiting the body's own defenses to provide protection, vaccines stand out as the most misunderstood of all interventions available in modern medicine. In a growing and influential worldwide subculture, vaccines are routinely maligned, demonized, and subjected to unrelenting disinformation campaigns.

In a survey by Dr. Sharma's hospital, more than half of 600 residents polled in the greater New York City metropolitan area said they do not want to get vaccinated against COVID-19. Their refusal is surprising in a city that registered more deaths from the pandemic virus than any other in the country. Similar surveys have also shown large percentages of people elsewhere in the United States turning thumbs down on CO-VID vaccination. A CDC study released in November 2020 found that 1 in 5 parents is vaccine hesitant. While medical experts attribute the growing rates of vaccine hesitancy to an active anti-vaccine movement, it remains a counterculture that's not likely to go away anytime soon. Like the proverbial genie, it can't be put back into the bottle, Sharma said.

74. How many COVID-19 vaccines exist?

While there are more than 200 COVID vaccines under study, not all have made it to human clinical research. By the end of 2020, only a handful had completed all three phases of randomized placebo-controlled clinical trials. Some Phase III trials, such as those for the innovative messenger RNA (mRNA) vaccines, have collectively involved tens of thousands of participants across the United States and around the world.

Dr. Anthony Fauci, director of the National Institute of Allergy and Infectious Diseases (NIAID), said in the early months of the pandemic that "finding a safe and effective vaccine to prevent infection with SARS-CoV-2

is an urgent public health priority." His agency collaborated with Moderna to produce their mRNA vaccine.
Two German biotechnology companies are also leaders
in mRNA vaccine development. But there are many
other types of vaccines under development in the
worldwide effort to beat back SARS-CoV-2. The chart
illustrates vaccines in use and those in development.

Institution(s)	Nation(s)	Vaccine Type
Altimmune	United States	Recombinant intranasal vaccine
Applied DNA Sciences, LinneaRx, Takis BioTech	United States	PCR-produced linear DNA vaccine
BioNTech, Pfizer	Germany, United States	mRNA (first in worldwide use)
Boston Children's Hospital	United States	Subunit vaccine plus adjuvants (for the elderly)
CanSino Biologics	China	Recombinant vaccine, Ad5nCoV (approved in China)
Codagenix, Serum Institute	United States, India	Live attenuated vaccine
CureVac	Germany	mRNA vaccine
Dyadic International	Israel	Recombinant vaccine plus monoclonal antibodies
Entos Pharmaceuticals	Canada	DNA vaccine
Generex	Canada	Peptide vaccine
GlaxoSmithKline, Clover Biopharmaceuticals	United States, China	Recombinant vaccine plus GSK adjuvants
Heat Biologics	United States	gp96 platform to produce viral antigens
INOVIO Pharmaceuticals	United States	DNA vaccine, INO-4800 (in a clinical trial)
Institut Pasteur, Themis Bioscience	France, Austria	SARS-CoV-2 antigen plus measles vector

Institution(s)	Nation(s)	Vaccine Type
Johnson & Johnson, Janssen Pharmaceuticals, Beth Israel Deaconess Medical Center	United States	Multiple candidate vaccines
Medicago	Canada	VLP (virus-like particle) vaccine
MIGAL Galilee Research Institute	Israel	IBV (infectious bronchitis vaccine)
Moderna Therapeutics, NIAID	United States	mRNA vaccine, mRNA 1273 (in worldwide use)
Novavax	United States	Nanoparticle vaccine
Oxford University, AstraZeneca	United Kingdom	Chimpanzee adenovirus-vectored vaccine, ChAdOx1 nCoV-19 (in use in Britain and approved by several other countries)
University of Pittsburgh	United States	Viral protein delivered by patch
University of Queensland	Australia	Molecular-clamp-processed vaccine
Regeneron Pharmaceuticals	United States	VelociSuite-produced antibodies
Sanofi	France	Recombinant DNA vaccine
Tonix Pharmaceuticals	United States	Vaccine utilizes horsepox platform
Vaxart	United States	Oral recombinant vaccine
Zydus Cadila	India	DNA vaccine and a live attenuated vaccine

75. What is an mRNA vaccine?

Messenger RNA (or mRNA) **vaccines** are a new concept in vaccinology. COVID-19 ushered in the era of mRNA vaccines because of the intense pressure scientists were under to produce vaccines to curb the global tide of pandemic infections. The emergence of effective mRNA vaccine technology is not only considered an important milestone in science, it is a breakthrough for managing coronaviruses in general. Vaccines were never developed for SARS or MERS, even though many attempts were made, and several efforts are still plod-dingly underway. Dr. Tal Zaks, chief medical officer at Moderna (one of the early developers of mRNA vaccine technology), told *Genetic Engineering and Biotechnology News* that mRNA vaccination offers some key benefits: "The potential advantage of an mRNA vaccine approach includes the ability to mimic natural infection [and] to stimulate a more potent immune response," Zaks said.

The speed at which these vaccines have been developed is astonishing. It took just 42 days from the time that scientists in China posted the complete genetic sequence of SARS-CoV-2 online in January of 2020 to the moment when Moderna's first mRNA dose was injected in a patient at Kaiser Permanente in Seattle, an early clinical testing site. In contrast, scientists worked for years, sometimes decades, to develop vaccines we now use routinely, such as the polio vaccine. The speed of modern vaccine development is in large part related to advances in molecular biology and genetics, enabling researchers to "take apart" a viral genome to see what makes it unique—but the basic science preceding the first mRNA vaccine began in the 1990s. The technology was pioneered by Ozlem Tureci and her husband Ugur Sahin, founders of the German biotech firm, BioNTech.

In November 2020, the partnership between Pfizer and BioNTech reported findings of clinical testing in thousands of volunteers, which demonstrated that its mRNA vaccine is 95% effective at preventing symptomatic COVID-19. Such extraordinarily high efficacy compares with that of the measles vaccine. The two-dose mRNA shot stimulates a robust immune response.

The Pfizer/BioNTech mRNA vaccine is made by artificially creating an mRNA sequence in the lab. Once injected into muscle cells, the sequence instructs the

Messenger RNA vaccine

A new type of vaccine that protects against infectious diseases. With just a single strand of mRNA, the vaccine teaches our cells to make a specific protein that triggers an immune response: The production of antibodies. If exposed to the actual virus, antibodies specific to it can destroy it. mRNA vaccines are up to 95% efficacious.

recipient's own cells to string together the precise order of amino acids that recreates the coronavirus' spike protein. The immune system learns to fight that protein because the sequence essentially says "foreign and possibly dangerous." This in turn causes the immune system to do two things: (1) mount an antibody response, and (2) form a memory of the foreign protein sequence to alert immune cells to attack it should it be encountered in the future.

The Pfizer/BioNTech vaccine was in development at the same time as other mRNA immunizations. The Moderna mRNA vaccine and a domestic German product all function similarly in the body. The Pfizer/BioNTech vaccine is a 30 microgram shot followed by a second dose of the same amount 21 days later. Moderna is a 100-microgram immunization followed by a booster of the same dosage 28 days later.

Moderna Therapeutics' mRNA-1273 vaccine was developed in collaboration with NIAID, which is led by Dr. Fauci. It was targeted early in its development for financing under the auspices of Operation Warp Speed, a Trump-era COVID-19 response project. The mRNA vaccine Pfizer developed with its German partner was not financed by this program. Moderna, however, also received funding from CEPI, the Coalition for Epidemic Preparedness Innovations, an Oslo, Norway-based nonprofit. The Moderna vaccine is 94.1% efficacious, comparable to Pfizer/BioNTech.

Globally, there is a third mRNA vaccine, which was developed by drug maker CureVac in Tübingen, Germany. There, Thorsten Schüller said his company's mRNA vaccine is not the first it had ever made. Prior to its work on an mRNA vaccine against SARS-CoV-2, it developed one for rabies.

Moderna's COVID-19 vaccine, like Pfizer's, was tested in thousands of clinical trial volunteers. The Moderna and NIAID researchers sought a diverse population to be part of clinical testing. An estimated 7,000 people throughout the United States who were 65 or older, and another 5,000 who were under 65 but had chronic health conditions, such as type 2 diabetes or severe obesity, were enrolled in clinical testing. High-risk groups made up 42% of clinical trial participants to ensure the vaccine was widely tested in a population that was as diverse as possible. All told, more than 30,000 people were part of the clinical trial. Moderna's vaccine also is more than 90% effective.

As with the Pfizer/BioNTech mRNA vaccine, the Moderna product has no viral components, but a simple mRNA "transcript," a sequence of genetic coding. For the Moderna vaccine, the mRNA sequence carries the code for a "prefusion spike protein." You may recall from Part 1, Question 2, that the spike protein is the business end of the virus—the protrusion that allows SARS-CoV-2 to connect with a human cell and begin the infection process. **Prefusion** simply means the conformation of the spike before it undergoes structural rearrangement as it latches onto the ACE2 receptor on the surface of human cells in the respiratory tract.

Prefusion

In virology, the shape of a spike protein before it latches onto the receptor that allows it to invade the cell.

As an analogy, think of an airplane approaching a runway for landing. When the plane is in the air, its wheels are folded into the aircraft's body, but as it makes its approach for landing, the wheels move into a different conformation, allowing the aircraft to touch down and roll along the runway. The viral spikes are in one conformation before it infects the cell and another afterward.

Messenger RNA vaccines have some advantages, but there are drawbacks as well. The Pfizer/BioNTech vaccine must be stored at an unworldly subzero temperature to maintain stability. This requirement can make use challenging in regions lacking ultracold freezers capable of sustaining vaccine vials at minus 94 degrees Fahrenheit. Moderna's vaccine must be stored at minus 4 degrees Fahrenheit, a temperature that makes its use more practical.

76. If there are mRNA vaccines, do DNA vaccines exist?

Yes, there are. DNA vaccines preceded mRNA vaccines by more than 20 years.

Dr. David B. Weiner, the molecular immunologist who directs the Wistar Institute's Vaccine and Immunology Center in Philadelphia, conducted research in the 1990s that laid the foundation for exploiting DNA's versatility for a vaccine.

DNA vaccines are designed by computer, Weiner explained, molecule by molecule, nothing is left to chance. The vaccines are double-stranded plasmids (small, circular DNA strands). Composing each segment is like fitting together LEGOs, Weiner said of producing a DNA vaccine.

Genomic vaccines

Vaccines composed of genetic sequences from DNA or RNA.

Both mRNA and DNA vaccines are known as **genomic vaccines** because they are composed of genetic sequences. In the early rush to determine which types of vaccines could help rein in the fast-moving pandemic, mRNA and DNA vaccines were high on the list of the CEPI, the Oslo-based nonprofit, which helps advance vaccine research.

Weiner, in an interview with *Genetic Engineering and Biotechnology News*, said CEPI chose to fund vaccine "technologies designed for rapid deployment." He added: "All of these technologies were chosen because they are fast and have conceptual advantages."

A vaccine based on Weiner's discoveries has been produced by INOVIO Pharmaceuticals in Plymouth Meeting, Pennsylvania. Like Moderna, INOVIO was among the first to get its vaccine into human clinical trials. Tests of the INOVIO vaccine, which is known as INO-4800, were conducted in the United States, South Korea, and China.

Weiner defined the race to develop vaccines against SARS-CoV-2 vaccines as the 21st century's equivalent to the Manhattan Project—the World War II-era program to harness atomic energy. "We are all in this together," Weiner said of the vaccine research, emphasizing that while it's a race, it's not a competition.

77. Why were COVID-19 vaccine trials suspended?

A different kind of COVID-19 vaccine was developed jointly by Oxford University's Jenner Institute and Oxford Vaccine Group in partnership with the pharmaceutical giant, AstraZeneca. This vaccine made the news when its clinical trial was temporarily suspended.

The vaccine, which is dubbed AZD12 (and also known during clinical trials as ChAdOx1 nCoV-19), differs from the mRNA and DNA vaccines developed in the United States and Germany. It has two key segments: One is a modified adenovirus, a common cold virus that causes the illness in chimpanzees. The virus is treated so that it is not infectious. Oxford refers to it as "a replication-deficient chimpanzee viral vector." As a vector, the adenovirus carries the genetic material of SARS-CoV-2's spike protein (which is the second segment) and delivers it into the body. After vaccination, the viral spike protein primes the immune system to attack SARS-CoV-2 if it later infects the body.

The clinical trial was not without a few problems. It was paused globally after a woman became ill during the clinical trial. The trial participant is said to have developed symptoms consistent with transverse myelitis, a rare inflammation of the spinal cord. A few weeks later, a 28-year-old man in Brazil, who was a participant in that country's arm of the research, died following a stroke. It was later reported that the man was in the placebo portion of the trial and did not receive the vaccine, so his stroke wasn't related to the vaccine itself. The vaccine is said to have a high level of efficacy and was approved for use in the United Kingdom and several other countries. It is less expensive than the mRNA vaccines and does not require special, ultracold maintenance.

Johnson & Johnson also briefly suspended a Phase III clinical trial for one of its vaccine candidates, JNJ-78436735, when one of its 60,000 volunteers developed a serious, unexplained illness during the trial. In November 2020, the company received $454 million in additional federal funding to support its massive clinical trial. Earlier in 2020, the company had received more than $1 billion in federal dollars. Johnson & Johnson's vaccine is a single-dose preparation, which is simpler than the two-dose regimens developed by the Pfizer/BioNTech partnership and Moderna.

78. Can the tuberculosis vaccine prevent COVID-19?

Bacille Calmette-Guérin (BCG)

A 100-year-old vaccine for tuberculosis that is being studied for effectiveness against COVID-19.

Countries that routinely administer the century-old tuberculosis vaccine, **Bacille Calmette-Guérin**, known as BCG, generally have lower incidence and/or mortality of COVID-19, according to anecdotal evidence. The vaccine is administered because these countries tend to have relatively high rates of tuberculosis. While large-scale randomized, placebo-controlled trials have not rigorously tested this observation, small epidemiological studies have been compelling. In one statistical study, for example, scientists have found that countries with mandatory BCG vaccination tended to have lower infection and death rates during the first 30 days of a COVID-19 outbreak.

Other research has shown that in Eastern European nations and countries such as India where BCG is still widely administered, mortality and COVID-19 severity have been lower compared with Western Europe or the United States, where the vaccine is not widely used. BCG is estimated to be about 70% to 80% effective in preventing tuberculosis, according to a report by the Gavi Vaccine Alliance.

TB in humans is caused by the bacterium *Mycobacterium tuberculosis*. BCG is a live, attenuated vaccine that uses a weakened version of a related bacterium, *Mycobacterium bovis*, to prevent tuberculosis and other mycobacterial infections. The vaccine was developed over a 13-year period between 1908 and 1921 by French bacteriologists Albert Calmette and Camille Guérin, who named the bacillus vaccine (*bacille* in French) after themselves. It remains the only TB vaccine approved in the United States and most of the rest of the world. Scientists theorize that it can stimulate a potent immune response not only against TB, but also against other infectious agents and even cancer. The vaccine is widely used in the treatment of bladder cancer.

BCG isn't the only existing vaccine that has raised scientific interest since the emergence of SARS-CoV-2. Dr. Robert Gallo, the noted HIV researcher and co-discoverer of the human immunodeficiency virus, has broached the possibility that the Sabin oral polio vaccine might be repurposed as a coronavirus preventive. In a letter to *The New York Times*, Gallo wrote that repurposing old vaccines for new applications isn't a novel concept.

"This might be done by using an approach that has worked against other viruses for years: simply feeding another virus to stimulate the body's innate immune system, ideally the Sabin oral polio vaccine (OPV), which is extremely safe, available, inexpensive and a powerful stimulant of an immediate, emergency response against a wide range of other viruses beyond polio," Gallo asserted. Such "repurposing" could have important potential upsides: Cost and safety. Developing new vaccines is expensive and time consuming, and that's without considering the cost (in both money and time) of producing enough doses for the millions upon millions of people who'll need it—both BCG and the Sabin polio vaccine have proven safety records and are relatively easy and cheap to produce.

So while we don't yet know for sure if BCG or other older vaccines work against COVID-19, there is good reason to keep investigating, if only as a stop-gap until more targeted vaccines can be widely distributed.

79. What is an antibody cocktail? Is it a vaccine?

Antibody cocktail

Lab-created monoclonal antibodies based on potent natural antibodies that have been selected for their robust activity.

An **antibody cocktail** is not a vaccine, but lab-created antibodies—monoclonal antibodies—that are based on potent natural antibodies targeted for their robust activity. Biotechnology innovator Regeneron Pharmaceuticals in New York and drug maker Eli Lilly in Indiana have developed cocktails made up of at least two monoclonal antibodies for the treatment of COVID-19. The antibodies are infused into patients, but do not produce ideal results in advanced COVID disease. The Regeneron product, REGN-COV2, was made famous when Donald Trump announced that he had been given the cocktail to treat his SARS-CoV-2 infection in early October 2020. Use of the Eli Lilly product in human testing, bamlanivimab, was briefly suspended for safety reasons, but in November 2020 it was granted an emergency use authorization by the FDA for people over age 12 who had mild to moderate COVID-19. The aim is to use the antibody preparation as a way to prevent these patients from becoming severely ill.

It's also important to note that the two COVID-19 monoclonal antibody products are not the first antibody cocktails for a serious viral infection. The FDA approved another monoclonal antibody cocktail, also made by Regeneron Pharmaceuticals, as an Ebola therapeutic in October 2020; this drug goes by the name Inmazeb (previously known as REGN-EB3). It is a combination of three monoclonal antibodies that target a glycoprotein on the surface of the Ebola virus. This Ebola glycoprotein can attach to human cells, enabling the virus to enter, but the cocktail of antibodies attaches to the protein and stops the infection process.

80. Is convalescent plasma a solution to COVID-19?

Convalescent plasma was a breakthrough treatment at the turn of the 20th century and won a Nobel Prize for Emil von Behring in the pre-antibiotic era. It is still useful today, and many hospitals solicit patients who have recovered from COVID-19 to donate their plasma.

Convalescent plasma

A straw-colored liquid portion of blood drawn from donors who have recovered from an infectious disease.

Convalescent plasma is the straw-colored liquid portion of blood drawn from donors who have recovered from an infectious disease. It has been used in the treatment of polio, influenza, Ebola, hepatitis, and many other infectious diseases. Antibodies collect in the plasma portion of blood, which is transfused into patients. The hope is that antibodies in the plasma will neutralize the virus and lead to a full recovery. The FDA has authorized convalescent plasma therapy for people with COVID-19. Studies of the therapy have had mixed results.

81. Are antibodies from llamas a treatment for COVID-19?

The hunt for an effective treatment for COVID-19 has led scientists down dozens of blind alleys, but llamas have turned out to be an unsuspected ally. The animals have particularly potent antibodies, and even fragments of their antibodies—nanobodies—produce a robust response against SARS-CoV-2 as well, laboratory studies have demonstrated.

Research by scientists at the University of Texas at Austin, the National Institutes of Health, and Ghent University in Belgium were in the vanguard of medical investigations examining llama antibodies in the fight against the pandemic coronavirus. The animals' antibodies neutralize SARS-CoV-2. The initial collaborative research has led to several other labs investigating llama antibodies. These antibodies are not yet ready for human clinical trials, but scientists suspect that in the not-too-distant future, llama antibodies will be the basis for therapeutics to treat infectious diseases, particularly COVID-19.

82. What is remdesivir, and how does it work?

Remdesivir is an antiviral medication that has been administered against a wide range of viral infections, often with lackluster results. It was approved by the FDA in October 2020 for use in adults and pediatric patients for treatment of COVID-19 and is sold under the brand name Veklury. Remdesivir is a product of Gilead Sciences, a California drug maker that had been testing the drug in patients infected with the Ebola virus.

Long before the drug was tested as a coronavirus therapeutic, it was tried in an array of viral infections. It was originally developed to target hepatitis C and a respiratory virus that circulates in winter known as respiratory syncytial virus (RSV). Remdesivir wasn't an effective treatment for either infectious disease, and a WHO-sponsored study revealed that it was only moderately effective against SARS-CoV-2.

However, a study that was funded by the National Institute of Allergy and Infectious Diseases (NIAID) and reported in an October 2020 issue of the *New England Journal of Medicine (NEJM)* showed that remdesivir shortened recovery time for patients hospitalized with COVID-19. The conclusion was based on findings from the completed Adaptive COVID-19 Treatment Trial (ACTT-1). But WHO issued a conditional recommendation in November 2020 against using the antiviral drug in hospitalized patients regardless of COVID severity. Based on research the agency sponsored, there is no evidence "that remdesivir improves survival and other outcomes." The conclusion was drawn by a WHO international guideline group.

It's believed that remdesivir works by blocking SARS-CoV-2's RNA polymerase, a key enzyme the virus uses to replicate its genetic material (RNA) and proliferate in human cells. The reason remdesivir was drafted into the COVID-19 armamentarium in the first place is because laboratory studies "suggested [it] was effective against viruses in the coronavirus family, such as Middle East Respiratory Syndrome (MERS) and Severe Acute Respiratory Syndrome (SARS)," according to an NIAID report. Even though doctors have administered remdesivir to patients during several Ebola outbreaks, the drug has not yet been approved for the infection.

83. Is wearing a mask equivalent to being vaccinated?

A novel theory published in the *NEJM* suggests that masks can serve as a substitute for a vaccine. The authors, Dr. Monica Gandhi and Dr. George Rutherford, both on staff at the University of California, San Francisco, are specialists in infectious diseases, and they say the notion is not as farfetched as it may sound. When in the presence of someone infected with SARS-CoV-2, the mask becomes a shield, and therefore blocks the bulk of airborne particles that are launched aloft during conversation or other simple encounters. While it is provocative to compare a mask to a vaccine, studies have already demonstrated that in populations where people adhere to masking mandates during pandemics, lives are inevitably spared.

If a mask can function as a crude vaccine, how exactly would that work? Gandhi and Rutherford posit in their theory—and it remains largely a theory—that masking filters out airborne coronavirus droplets, limiting the amount of droplets that a person inhales if exposed. Only a few particles can breach a mask, the doctors say, but those particles are enough to alert the immune system—without supplying enough to make the mask-wearer sick.

A vaccine works similarly when people are immunized—they are exposed to only a small dose, just enough to spark an immune response. So, in theory, by filtering out most but not all vaccine particles, the mask itself is doing what a vaccine injection would do: Exposing the wearer to just enough virus to allow the immune system to respond without exposing them to so much virus that they develop the COVID-19 disease itself.

The theory has not been corroborated by rigorous research involving a population of people at average risk of infection in a pandemic. "If this theory bears out, population-wide masking, with any type of mask that increases acceptability and adherence, might contribute to increasing the proportion of SARS-CoV-2 infections that are asymptomatic," Gandhi and Rutherford wrote in their *NEJM* commentary.

Unfortunately, the Gandhi/Rutherford commentary arrived in the waning weeks of the Trump administration, which had fostered a climate of science denial and led to many people flouting the benefits of mask-wearing in general. Thus, even an easy and inexpensive method that *might* actually mimic the impact of a vaccine stood out as an object of contention. Not only were many people discouraged from masking up, some anti-maskers labeled face coverings infringements on their civil liberties. At the time of this writing, COVID-19 cases continued not only to surge throughout the United States, hospitals strained to cope with the explosive number of patients who were dying at a rate of 1 every 30 seconds as 2020 drew to a close.

PART EIGHT

Pandemic Preparedness: Quarantine and Virus Tracking

Why is pandemic planning important?

Has the COVID-19 pandemic produced lessons for future pandemic planning?

Is forced vaccination written into pandemic preparedness plans?

More . . .

84. Why is pandemic planning important?

Pandemic planning

Development of a strategy that anticipates the public health, medical, societal, and national security concerns that can arise during a pandemic.

Pandemic planning is centered on developing a strategy that anticipates the public health, medical, societal, and national security concerns that can arise during one of the most extraordinary infectious disease events to affect humankind: a pandemic.

Years before COVID-19 emerged, the Centers for Disease Control and Prevention had produced some of the most comprehensive, evidenced-based plans in the world crafted by top epidemiologists, policy experts, and scientists. These plans were ignored by the Trump administration, which rebuffed the computer model- ing studies, data on re-stocking the Strategic National Stockpile, and plans on how to keep the public well in- formed. Quietly, the administration had run pandemic preparedness exercises in 2019, which carried the code name Crimson Contagion a massive war games-style battle plan that involved several states. The exercises, which were led by the Department of Health and Human Services (HHS), occurred just months before COVID-19 erupted in real life. But any lessons that might have been learned from the experience were not implemented when the scenario became reality. (Crimson Contagion had an eerie resemblance to what actually happened, in that it postulated a pandemic virus, albeit an influenza virus, originating in China that was spread by international tourists.) In the event of a genuine outbreak, the CDC had prioritized keeping the states and the public informed as one of its core pandemic response aims. Additionally, the agency had well-laid plans to work aggressively toward containment by taking the following steps:

1. Ramping up surveillance to track the spread of a novel pathogen;

2. Developing containment measures with state and local health departments;

3. Regularly reporting transmission, prevalence, and mortality data to the public and providing the public with accurate information on preventive/protection measures;

4. Coordinating diagnostic testing and vaccine development and distribution;

5. Working with major international partners, such as the World Health Organization.

Despite the detailed plans of the United States government's public health authorities, the country spiraled downward into the worst mortality and highest number of positive coronavirus cases in the first year of the pandemic. Instead of containment, infections raged out of control. The United States fared worse than Brazil, Mexico, India, Russia, and South Africa. Despite the enormous resources of the United States, other countries had far better outcomes. Australia, Canada, and Germany were among the wealthy nations that approached the pandemic more strategically than the United States, and as a result, experienced rates of infection and death that, adjusted for population size, were substantially lower.

The devastating outcomes occurred largely because science-driven public health directives were shunted aside in favor of politicizing public health measures, deriding masks, downplaying the risk of the virus or comparing it to the flu. Because the Trump administration had hobbled the CDC early in the coronavirus pandemic, the public was never given a simple yet firm explanation of what a pandemic is and how it differs from viral infections that circulate seasonally.

Instead of the richest country in the world having the best outcomes, the best results occurred in much smaller countries with far fewer resources and bare-bones preparedness budgets.

Vietnam, Taiwan, Iceland, New Zealand, and Singapore moved to the front of the line.

1. In the first wave, **Vietnam** reported only 401 cases and zero deaths by instituting its emergency public health plan as soon as cases were reported in China.

2. **Taiwan** had 455 cases and seven deaths and, like Vietnam, instituted its emergency plan, which also called for closing its borders. The country began a massive testing and tracing program.

3. **Iceland** put its emergency disaster plan into effect to control the pandemic. The country reported 1,839 cases and 10 deaths as Trump administration members praised Sweden instead, citing its controversial attempt at instituting a "herd immunity" strategy even without a vaccine. By the close of 2020, Iceland had recorded fewer than 30 deaths, in comparison to over 6,400 in Sweden.

4. In **New Zealand**, 1,205 cases were recorded in the first wave and 22 people died. A testing and tracing program took effect and healthcare practitioners were required to report any suspected cases.

5. In **Singapore**, there were 48,434 cases but only 27 deaths. Borders were closed, aggressive testing and tracing went into effect, and a communication strategy that kept the public regularly informed helped limit the infection rate.

In the United States, the HHS, the agency that oversees the CDC, also has an Office of Global Affairs, which directs the Office of Pandemics and Emerging

Threats (PET). Alex Azar, head of HHS, hired as his chief of staff for pandemic affairs Brian Harrison, a man whose last job before signing on to work on one of the worst pandemics in a century was as a breeder of labradoodle dogs—not someone who had expertise in epidemiology or public health.

85. Has the COVID-19 pandemic produced lessons for future pandemic planning?

Studies conducted as the pandemic progressed have produced a flurry of leads on where people tend to congregate and how those places of human interaction affect coronavirus transmission. The data likely will have an impact on pandemic policies and future pandemic planning.

Tracking the movements of nearly 100 million people anonymously via their cell phones revealed that locations of high-density human interaction account for the locations where viral transmission is most likely to occur. People are extremely social animals, most gravitating to crowded spaces for food, drinks, conversation, sermons, and singing. Scientists eavesdropped regularly on legions of people to determine what types of activities and venues were driving the pandemic. No one was aware of being tracked, but the data spoke volumes. The unusual research has provided an illuminating framework to understand where (outside the home) the coronavirus is most frequently transmitted.

In a collaborative analysis, researchers from Stanford University and Northwestern University say restaurants, bars, gyms, cafes, hotels, and places of worship are sites where people are most likely to spread—and catch—SARS-CoV-2. People's homes, nevertheless, remain the number-one spot.

Jure Leskovec, writing in the journal *Nature*, reported on how cell phone data was used to track the movements of people in large U.S. cities—Los Angeles, Chicago, New York, Washington, D.C., and six other metropolitan areas—as they left their homes and traveled to more than 500,000 locations from March 1 to May 2, 2020. Geospatial data allowed the researchers to determine how long people stayed at each site, how often they visited it, and how crowded each venue was at the time of the visit. It smacks of espionage, but it was designed to help pandemic preparedness planners gain an understanding of how and where infections occur.

Leskovec and the team superimposed the geospatial data over a model of viral transmission to nail down specific patterns of infection. Although the research team could not tell whether the individuals they silently tracked actually became infected, their model answered the scientific questions about where they went, the frequency of visits, and whether crowds were present, which allowed them to predict infections in a given region. Moreover, the predicted infections matched caseloads tabulated in the targeted cities as represented in coronavirus tracking statistics compiled by *The New York Times*.

In Chicago, for example, the researchers discovered that just 10% of crowded sites accounted for 80% of real-life infections. And not all sites are equal as places where the coronavirus spreads. Chances of getting infected are high in coffee shops, gyms, and houses of worship, but the risks are about four times less likely than in restaurants and cafes.

Aside from the Stanford–Northwestern study, administrators of colleges and universities had argued early in the pandemic that maintaining physical distancing among college student is a difficult task. While it is possible to space students six feet or more apart in classrooms, these efforts are of little use once the students are out of class and on their own time. Weekends are especially trying, when restaurants, bars, gyms and other close-quarter venues beckon.

86. What is the Strategic National Stockpile?

The **Strategic National Stockpile** (SNS), created in 1999, is made up of tons of pharmaceuticals and medical supplies designed to meet the needs of a public health disaster.

Strategic National Stockpile
A group of large caches of emergency equipment maintained in secret locations throughout the United States.

The SNS is not a single entity but a group of large caches of emergency equipment maintained in secret locations throughout the United States. Having supplies in multiple locations makes it easier to quickly deploy equipment and supplies to sites in need. In the government's original wording, the SNS is described as "the nation's largest supply of lifesaving pharmaceuticals and medical supplies for use in a public health emergency severe enough to cause local supplies to run out."

The SNS includes medications, vaccines, and emergency supplies such as ventilators and personal protective equipment (PPE) for healthcare workers. PPE includes disposable medical gloves, gowns, one-piece coveralls, face shields, goggles, and surgical masks as well as N-95 respirator masks, which are capable of filtering out 95% of airborne particles, including viruses.

Jared Kushner, a White House adviser during the Trump administration and Donald Trump's son-in-law, changed the mission statement of the SNS in April 2020. From now on: "The Strategic National Stockpile's role is to supplement state and local supplies during public health emergencies," according to Kushner. The administration falsely claimed that it had inherited a depleted stockpile with empty shelves from the Obama administration, a charge vehemently denied by members of the Obama administration. A rare tour of an SNS facility by a reporter for National Public Radio, whose accompanying photos also allowed a glimpse inside the SNS in June of 2016, revealed a vast warehouse brimming with supplies to help medical professionals tend to public health in an emergency.

The stockpile is rarely used and is supposed to be frequently updated to maintain the quality of the equipment and to replace medications and vaccines that have expired.

In addition to rolling out supplies during the COVID-19 pandemic, the SNS has been tapped to aid victims of natural disasters, including the growing number of hurricanes that have occurred in recent years. In the past, supplies were deployed to aid people injured in the wake of the World Trade Center attacks in New York City on September 11, 2001.

The SNS will have to be restocked during the Biden administration to ensure that enough equipment is available to address ongoing and future coronavirus infections and other major emergencies.

87. Does a Biden administration portend a return to pandemic planning and evidenced-based public health?

From his first speech as president-elect to all speeches afterward, Joseph R. Biden, Jr., has promised that his administration will rely on scientific experts to guide the nation in major public health emergencies. His coronavirus task force is made up of leading experts in infectious and emerging diseases, global health, medicine, and public policy. One of his task force members, Dr. Michael Osterholm, an epidemiologist and director of the Center for Infectious Disease Research and Policy (CIDRAP), has been quoted as saying about the coronavirus pandemic: "I don't think we are going to see one, two, or three waves. I think we are going to see one very difficult forest fire of cases."

Biden's chief of staff, Ron Klain, was President Barack Obama's "Ebola czar," the bureaucrat who coordinated the U.S. response to the West African epidemic in 2014. Biden has been an advocate of a universal mask mandate as a method of blunting the explosive spread of the virus.

88. Is forced vaccination written into pandemic preparedness plans?

A cornerstone of pandemic planning is identifying the causative agent and developing a vaccine against it. While the federal government would likely never order mass vaccinations, state and local health department jurisdictions might recommend that certain groups consider vaccination, and certain employers, particularly those in the healthcare arena, might even require it.

There are precedents for a vaccine mandate. In 1905, a Supreme Court case, *Massachusetts v. Jacobsen*, set the legal precedent that public authorities do have the right to require healthy people to get vaccinated in circumstances where a serious and urgent health rationale exists, such as an epidemic. (The court did agree that people who had serious adverse reactions to vaccines or other health-related risk factors could not be forced to participate.)

During the 2009 H1N1 flu pandemic, the State of New York required healthcare workers to be vaccinated against both seasonal and H1N1 influenza. The demand didn't seem unreasonable given the State Department of Health's argument that being vaccinated would prevent the spread of the pandemic virus in hospitals and nursing homes. But many healthcare workers balked, and dozens protested and carried picket signs in the state capitol of Albany, demonstrating against the requirement.

Although many of the vaccine contrarians were registered nurses, who frequently recommended flu shots to patients, some argued against the shots because they were being required to get *two* influenza vaccines. Their opposition centered on skepticism about the H1N1 vaccine, which they claimed was new and had not been tested in a clinical trial. This concern was based on a misunderstanding of how "new" flu vaccines are produced. Unlike the vaccines created against COVID-19, some of which involve first-of-its-kind technology (see Questions 74 and 75), flu shots have been made in the U.S. since the 1940s, and when a new strain emerges, it is incorporated into vaccines using existing technology. At the time of the H1N1 pandemic, flu shots had been manufactured by way of the same egg-based technology that had been in use for nearly 70 years. Clinical trials were therefore not required because even though the H1N1 influenza strain might be "new," the formula used to manufacture the vaccine was not.

In contrast, the genomic COVID-19 immunizations, particularly the mRNA vaccines, have never been administered to people on a large scale—they're still new technology. Therefore, the mRNA vaccines required a randomized clinical trial to test their efficacy and safety compared against a placebo.

89. Are there any pandemic preparedness lessons from the 1918 influenza pandemic?

Some of the strategies that were employed in 1918 have been used in combat against SARS-CoV-2 in many countries as the coronavirus circumnavigated the globe: School and business closings; discouraging large gatherings; dissuading people from attending church services, and encouraging the use of masks. The difference between the early 20th century and the early 21st is that many of the strategies relied upon more than a century ago were ad hoc measures that public health officials instituted on the fly.

Medical authorities of the day were astute enough to realize that a pandemic virus is like a match burning through dry grass. The closures kept people out the virus's path and spared lives. Quarantine was an old-school standby that came in handy during an era when effective pharmaceuticals were nonexistent, and isolation prevented an infection's spread.

Some measures were crude and wouldn't make the grade in a modern world. So-called Mask Slackers—people who refused to don a mask—could be sent to jail in San Francisco for two weeks. In Chicago, sneezing in public could warrant arrest. New York City had its chain of islets in the East River—the quarantine islands—where those who flouted hygiene rules could find themselves isolated.

Yet as storied as that pandemic has become, there are many aspects about it that remain forever lost to history. Survivors didn't talk about it much after it tailed off in 1919. It was unlike the coronavirus pandemic in multiple ways. The respiratory infection mostly preyed on people in the prime of their lives—people age 18 to 40—and 100 million people of all ages succumbed worldwide during a point in history when the number of people on Earth was one-fourth the size of the global population today.

90. What is self-quarantine? Is that an old-school measure?

Anyone exposed to SARS-CoV-2 may be at risk of developing COVID-19, and therefore is advised by the CDC to "**self-quarantine**" for 10 days to avoid spreading the infection. As a method of preventing the infection of others, self-quarantine is more of a 20th-century strategy than a 21st-century idea, as it was used during outbreaks of measles, whooping cough, and scarlet fever in the era before vaccines. Dr. Lisa Lockerd Maragakis, a specialist in infectious diseases at Johns Hopkins University, reports that self-quarantine involves following:

Self-quarantine

The practice of voluntarily restricting oneself to one's home and avoiding all contact with other people for a two-week period to prevent spreading an infection.

- Practicing standard hygiene and washing hands frequently
- Not sharing things like towels and utensils
- Staying at home
- Not having visitors
- Staying at least 6 feet away from other people in your household

Once your quarantine period has ended, if you do not have symptoms, follow your doctor's instructions on how to return to your normal routine.

91. Does the U.S. government have "quarantine powers" to evaluate foreign visitors for potential pandemic infections?

The CDC's quarantine powers refer to the agency's efforts to keep highly contagious and emerging infections out of the country. Over the years, the agency has maintained the U.S. Quarantine Stations, which are located in airports and along land-border crossings nationwide. With a pandemic virus having arrived in January of 2020, the question is, could it have been stopped?

Many experts, ranging from those at Johns Hopkins University to scientists at the CDC, say the answer is probably no. One of the key characteristics of SARS-CoV-2 infections is the large percentage of people who are asymptomatic. It would have been impossible for Quarantine Station personnel to know if someone onboard an international flight was infected with a potentially deadly virus unless flight attendants on the aircraft recognized the passenger was ailing.

Even though the pandemic virus was missed on arrival (probably having come into the country via more than one asymptomatic passenger), that doesn't mean the stations aren't worthwhile. Even though the pandemic virus slipped into the United States, the 20 stations located around the country remain integral to the nation's pandemic disease defense. For example, when an international flight lands with a sick passenger, health officers from a U.S. Quarantine Station have legal authority to evaluate the individual.

Officers are trained in the diagnosis of exotic infections and also possess legal authority to detain a passenger with unusual symptoms. A sick passenger would be kept in the station only long enough for a thorough medical evaluation before being released or sent to an isolation unit at a hospital.

When a pandemic occurs, the network of quarantine stations is expected to play a key role acting as a firewall to keep the infection out of the United States. The stations are not, however, equipped to isolate entire planeloads of passengers.

92. I don't remember masks or social distancing ever being recommended. Is this new to pandemic preparedness?

Masks and social distancing have been mandated on multiple occasions in other parts of the world. They were mandated in the United States during the 1918 flu pandemic and were prominent among the measures that helped defeat SARS globally in 2004.

Masks form a blockade preventing the inhalation of viral particles that can be exhaled or coughed into the surrounding environment from someone nearby, or during conversation. Dr. Leana Wen, a visiting professor of Health Policy and Management at George Washington University in Washington, D.C., has emphasized that masks are among the most potent tools that most people have available. "Actually, masks save lives. You can reduce transmission by more than 70%. If people wear masks, they protect the person wearing the mask as well as everyone else around that person as well."

93. Are coronaviruses the only types of infectious agents likely to cause pandemics now that COVID-19 has emerged?

Numerous viruses, some that have yet to be identified by scientists can lead to a pandemic. Mindful of this possibility, virus trackers are scouring rainforests, bat caves, rat warrens, pig pens, and birds' nests for exotic pathogens that might trigger the next pandemic.

COVID-19 wasn't the only deadly infectious disease to emerge in 2019 (see Question 94). Just because the world was waylaid by the worst pandemic in a century doesn't mean that other viruses aren't lurking in the wild. Avian flu viruses are still a potential threat, which is why surveillance remains one of the most important activities that governments can fund.

94. Is surveillance for potential pandemic viruses a way to stop pandemics before they start?

One of the most important activities that public health agencies in this country—and beyond—can fund is surveillance for emerging pathogens around the world. The first of the three lethal coronaviruses that emerged in the 21st century took experts in infectious diseases by surprise, but after reviewing the evidence, scientists predicted that more would follow. And even though the COVID-19 pandemic is the most explosive pandemic in a century, it won't be the last. Scientists, nevertheless, say it's possible to blunt the forces that lead to zoonotic pandemics by stopping the human activities that bring people inexorably into contact with wildlife.

We are constantly confronted by newly emerging viruses. Case in point: The novel coronavirus that emerged in Wuhan, China, in 2019 wasn't the only deadly pathogen to cause an outbreak that year. A much smaller, but far deadlier, rodent-borne Ebola-like hemorrhagic virus infected people in Bolivia.

Scientists call that infectious agent the Chapare virus, named after Bolivia's Chapare region, located more than 350 miles east of La Paz, the country's capital. Virus trackers say Chapare is more lethal than SARS-CoV-2, killing about three in every five people who contract it. It causes infection when humans come into contact with rat urine or feces. Although the virus doesn't appear to pose a threat to people in the United States, no one knows with certainty what may happen in the future.

As with bats, rodents are a source of viruses that don't kill the host animals but pose a lethal threat to humans. Chapare can be passed from one person to another, a first step among viruses that can cause community outbreaks. Chapare was first identified in 2004, but it has not gone away.

That's why surveillance of viruses in the wild is important: Virtually any species can be the source of a future pandemic virus. Just as bats are carriers of betacoronaviruses, the category of coronavirus that causes the human diseases SARS, MERS, and COVID-19, some rodents also harbor this category of coronavirus.

Bats, nevertheless, remain a worrisome source of infectious agents, and some bat species in many parts of the world are becoming more comfortable in human environments. A combination of human-inflicted deforestation and climate change alter the bats' habitats forever, and that forces them into closer contact with people, providing an opportunity for viruses the bats carry—often without any harm to the bats—to transfer to humans.

PART NINE

Guarding Your Health

Is it a good idea to consider getting vaccinated against COVID-19?

How can you tell if "health" information is disinformation? Is disinformation dangerous?

What is the right way to wear a mask?

More . . .

95. Is it a good idea to consider getting vaccinated against COVID-19?

Vaccination is a proven method of reducing personal risk as well as eliminating epidemics in communities. Being immunized also lowers the potential for long-term disease-associated disability and death.

Yet even though vaccination is a personal decision, it is also one with public health implications, especially in a pandemic, because a pandemic virus affects vast numbers of people. Your decision to vaccinate or not vaccinate can have an impact beyond yourself. By choosing to vaccinate, you are one less link in what theoretically could become a chain of transmission.

With that in mind, each individual has to ask whether they're willing to endure the consequences if they refuse to get immunized, but wind up becoming infected.

Lessons abound from throughout history about the important role vaccination has played in controlling devastating infectious diseases. Herd immunity (see Question 24), which is achieved through vaccination, has eliminated the threats of measles, mumps, rubella, and other so-called childhood diseases in much of the developed world. However, the **vaccine hesitancy movement** in recent decades has caused old foes, such as measles, to re-emerge in many developed countries, including surprising hot spots throughout the United States in recent years.

Vaccine hesitancy movement

A belief system based on misinformation that advocates shunning vaccination. The main tenet of "anti-vaxxers" is that vaccines are dangerous to health.

The WHO notes that vaccine "scares" receive more public attention than vaccination effectiveness, even though "independent experts and WHO have shown that vaccines are far safer than therapeutic medicines," according to a report by the agency.

On the whole, vaccines have an excellent safety record and most vaccine scares have been shown to be false alarms. The leading U.S. and European vaccines developed to prevent COVID-19 have undergone extensive testing in clinical trials that have studied tens of thousands of people, including those in high-risk groups and people of advanced ages.

96. How can you tell if "health information" is disinformation? Is disinformation dangerous?

Pandemics, as it turns out, are episodes when disinformation flourishes wildly, almost keeping pace with the spread of the virus itself. Disinformation and conspiracy theories have no sources, no data, and usually take the form of wild claims about health issues. Such claims travel by social media and word-of-mouth, sometimes seeming to have an air of legitimacy.

One widespread claim against masks that circulated on social media asserted that face coverings cause staph (bacterial) infections. The claim is incorrect and most likely had roots in the extensive anti-masker community that considered mask mandates an affront to their civil liberties.

Other wild claims can be traced directly to political sources. Disinformation was spread by Donald Trump, Jr., who claimed that deaths due to COVID-10 were overinflated—which was a conspiracy theory circulated by the fringe QAnon group based on a false interpretation of CDC data. According to the fact-checking website FactCheck.org, the CDC had explained in the footnote to its weekly COVID-19 mortality update that the chart "shows the types of health conditions and contributing causes mentioned in conjunction with deaths involving coronavirus disease 2019 (COVID-19). For 6% of the deaths, COVID-19 was the only cause mentioned." Individuals seized on this figure and used it to falsely claim only 6% of victims had actually died of COVID-19 and insisted that all other deaths should be attributed to other conditions, like heart disease or diabetes, which the patient had before being infected. This suggestion is based on a misunderstanding—either a deliberate one or out of sheer ignorance. A person with comorbidities who gets COVID-19 may be at higher risk of death because of those comorbidities, but it's still the COVID-19 infection that caused the death. Put another way: Would that patient have died at this time *without* COVID-19? If the answer to that question is *no*, or even *probably not*, then COVID-19 is the **proximate cause**, meaning, the most immediate determining factor that caused the death. There may be other contributing factors, but the proximate cause is the "tipping point."

Proximate cause

The most immediate factor leading to an outcome.

Donald Trump, Jr.'s remarks dovetailed with claims by his father that doctors profited each time they listed COVID as the reason for a patient's demise on death certificates. This is also untrue; medical billing codes note diagnoses and complicating factors, but the cost of services billed to a patient, and insurer, or Medicaid/Medicare is determined by what services were provided to the patient and by whom, not by what caused the patient's death. This disinformation from father and son was clearly aimed at distracting the public from the sweeping pandemic and the exponential growth in cases and deaths. The two claims were made as the number of cases soared past the 9 million mark and the number of deaths was heading north to a quarter million.

Nowhere was disinformation more evident than at the Sturgis Motorcycle Rally, which ran from August 7 to 16, 2020, in Sturgis, South Dakota. The annual rally attracts bikers from throughout the United States. The belief that COVID-19 is equivalent to seasonal flu and that face masks infringe on civil liberties were two key lines of disinformation that allowed many attendees to laugh off masking and flout social distancing during the event. News footage showed bikers in bars, tattoo parlors, restaurants, and other venues. Some bikers who were interviewed by reporters said they had no fear of contracting COVID-19. Several explained that news stories about the pandemic were overblown.

Yet within weeks of the gathering—attended by 500,000 bikers—cases in South Dakota and other midwestern states spiked. One study from researchers at San Diego State University estimated that the potential worst-case scenario for virus transmission was 266,000 cases. The study examined cell phone data allowing researchers to trace the movements of nonresidents in Sturgis, pinpointing where they went during the rally and where they dispersed after they left. They then used these data to model how many people might come into contact with the 500,000 attendees and estimate potential virus transmission rates to determine how many cases might be generated by the rally.

Although it's impossible to determine if the San Diego scientists' prediction is correct, data from multiple sources suggest the rally was among a number of problems that led to a troubling explosion of cases throughout the midwest following the massive gathering.

The governor of South Dakota, Kristi Noem, lambasted the scientific findings as fiction, but her policies helped seed a burdensome COVID caseload that strained her state's healthcare system for weeks.

Noem allowed the rally to occur in the first place, and her longstanding anti-mask stance grew out of the conspiracy theory that face coverings were of dubious value. By the fall of 2020 the number of cases and hospitalizations in the state were so overwhelming, the South Dakota State Medical Association was pleading with the public to wear masks. "To show respect and passion for physicians and other frontline health providers and everyone in our communities, the South Dakota State Medical Association (SDSMA) urges South Dakotans to help preserve our healthcare workforce ... The SDSMA supports masking and will continue to plead with the public to wear face masks in public."

The association pointed to the extraordinary strain that COVID-19 cases were having on South Dakota hospitals and their staffs. The test positivity rate for South Dakota was 44.1% in mid November, according to Becker's Hospital Review, a rate that placed the state second in the nation for an exceptionally high test positivity rate. The Mayo Clinic defines the test positivity rate as the percentage of coronavirus tests that are positive for the virus out of the total number of coronavirus tests performed to date. At the time, only Wyoming ranked higher at 58.9. New York City's test positivity rate had hit 3.0 around the same time and the mayor announced school closures.

Even though 266,000 Sturgis-related cases remains questionable, the test positivity rate in the aftermath of the rally is not in question, nor are the pleas of the South Dakota State Medical Association.

What got lost in the argument over numbers is this: the San Diego research uncovered a superspreading event fed by disinformation that impacted public health. Both South and North Dakota as well as Wyoming, Wisconsin, Michigan and Iowa became focal points of infection as a devastating autumn wave of COVID-19 swept across the country. Bikers had come from those states and beyond. Precisely how much of the problem was caused by people believing disinformation is yet another unknown.

Numerous studies have found that believing disinformation can adversely affect human behavior. To avoid disinformation, it is imperative to seek information from authoritative research. Here are 10 excellent, reliable sources to use when seeking information about COVID-19 and coronaviruses in general:

1. The Johns Hopkins University's Coronavirus Resource Center (https://coronavirus.jhu.edu/)
2. The Mayo Clinic's COVID-19 resource page (https://www.mayoclinic.org/coronavirus -covid-19)
3. National Institute of Allergy and Infectious Diseases COVID-19 resources (https://www .niaid.nih.gov/research/covid-19-resources)
4. Centers for Disease Control and Prevention Coronavirus (COVID-19) resource page (https://www.cdc.gov/coronavirus/2019-ncov /index.html)
5. University of Washington's Institute for Health Metrics and Evaluation COVID-19 resource (http://www.healthdata.org/covid)

6. Infectious Diseases Society of America's Real-Time COVID-19 Learning Network (https://www.idsociety.org/covid-19-real-time-learning-network/)

7. American Public Health Association's COVID-Guidance (https://www.apha.org/topics-and-issues/communicable-disease/coronavirus/guidance)

8. Center for Infectious Disease Research and Policy (CIDRAP) at the University of Minnesota: Novel Coronavirus (COVID-19) Resource Center (https://www.cidrap.umn.edu/covid-19)

9. World Health Organization: Coronavirus disease (COVID-19) pandemic (https://www.who.int/emergencies/diseases/novel-coronavirus-2019)

10. Association of State and Territorial Health Officials COVID-19 page (https://www.astho.org/COVID-19/)

97. What is the right way to wear a mask?

A mask should cover your face from the bridge of the nose and extend to underneath your chin. It should feel comfortable to wear and never should be pulled down under your chin to talk. While experts recommend that a mask should feel secure, it should not be tight, and you should be able to talk through it. You should not touch your mask while it is on your face, and you should avoid touching masks being worn by children as well.

It is recommended by public health experts at Johns Hopkins University that you should wash your hands before donning your mask and after touching it. You should touch your mask only by its bands or ties when putting it on or taking it off, according to the Johns Hopkins advice.

Reusable masks should be washed after each time they're worn.

98. Are masks with air valves a good choice?

Although many people wear masks in public to guard against the coronavirus, those with exhalation valves are considered ineffective and may promote the spread of infection. It is important to know which masks to avoid thinking that you're protected when in actuality you are not. Mutations have increased the contagiousness of SARS-CoV-2 with the emergence of variants, such as B.1.1.7, first identified in the United Kingdom in November 2020. By January 2021, the variant had spread to more than 30 countries, including the United States. Another SARS-CoV-2 variant that evolved in South Africa, E484K, also is noteworthy for its contagiousness. The mutations identified in the South African variant are in the spike protein, but differ from the mutations found in B.1.1.7. Current vaccines can help the body mount an effective immune response, but masks remain an important line of defense. A key to guarding your health in a pandemic is to choose an effective mask.

The National Institute of Standards and Technology (NIST) conducted a study of masks with exhalation valves and found they allow exhaled air to exit in fairly large streams without the benefit of filtering. Exhaled air from cloth masks is filtered as the wearer breathes. N-95 masks are among the best options because exceptionally minuscule viral particles cannot breach the mask's materials, which is why they're worn by healthcare professionals and essential workers. Valved masks defeat the purpose of wearing a mask, the NIST concluded.

NIST is a physical sciences laboratory of the U.S. Department of Commerce. As part of its research on valved masks, scientists at the laboratory produced a video with a split screen showing a man wearing a mask with a valve alongside a man wearing an N-95 mask. A large stream of air is seen being released from the valve as the man in the valved mask exhales. In contrast, the exhaled air from the man in the N-95 is filtered, producing a barely visible cloud of expelled air.

99. What is cough hygiene? What is hand hygiene?

Cough hygiene

The practice of covering your mouth when you cough to limit the spread of airborne viruses.

Cough hygiene is probably something your parents cautioned you about many times as a child, but of course, they very likely didn't use the arcane "cough hygiene" terminology, or its equally obtuse cousin, "cough etiquette." The terms simply mean the practice of covering your mouth when you cough. This is important advice wherever you are—at home, school, at a restaurant, or in the workplace, because inattention to how you cough can result in many people around you getting sick, especially if you are asymptomatically infected with SARS-CoV-2.

If you are curious about the basics of "Cough Etiquette 101," here are a few tips:

1. Cover your nose and mouth with a tissue every time you cough, and appropriately dispose the tissue.
2. If you do not have a tissue, cough into your sleeve at the elbow. Do not use your hand to cover your mouth.
3. Always wash your hands after coughing, even if you coughed into your sleeve.
4. Stay home when you feel sick.

Hand hygiene refers to a way of cleaning one's hands to substantially reduce the presence of pathogens to avoid getting sick or spreading infection to others. Although the name sounds stilted, it simply means frequent, thorough handwashing.

Hand hygiene
The practice of using frequent, thorough handwashing to prevent the spread of diseases.

Soap is an enveloped virus's worst enemy because it breaks them apart. This is good news, because even though SARS-CoV-2 is largely thought of as a virus that is transmitted through the air when someone talks, coughs, sneezes, or breathes, there is a chance that it can be transferred from someone's hands to frequently touched surfaces.

Indeed, according to the CDC, pathogens of any kind can contaminate surfaces and cause infections when you do any of the following:

- Touch your eyes, nose, and mouth with unwashed hands
- Eat with unwashed hands
- Blow your nose, cough, or sneeze into hands and then touch other people's hands or common objects

183

The WHO contends that people do not always wash their hands properly. The areas most frequently missed, the agency has found, are the thumbs and the back of each hand and the tips of the fingers. Most people also do not spend enough time washing their hands. The CDC recommends following these steps to ensure that your hands are properly washed:

1. Wet your hands with clean, running water (warm or cold), turn off the tap, and apply soap.
2. Lather your hands by rubbing them together with the soap. Lather the back of your hands, between your fingers, and under your nails.
3. Scrub your hands for at least 20 seconds. Need a timer? Hum the "Happy Birthday" song from beginning to end twice.
4. Rinse your hands well under running water.
5. Dry your hands using a clean towel.

While washing with soap and water is best, an alcohol-based hand sanitizer that contains at least 60% alcohol is an appropriate substitute.

100. Is having a family pandemic plan a good idea?

Most people did not have a personal pandemic plan when COVID-19 hit the United States in the early months of 2020. Scenes on television news, the Internet, and in newspapers of people buying insane amounts of toilet paper illuminated what constituted a pandemic plan for many in the United States.

The CIDRAP at the University of Minnesota developed a personal pandemic plan for pandemic flu, which works well for any type of pathogen that causes casualties and confines people to their homes.

Here are some of CIDRAP's suggestions:

Planning for a pandemic:

1. Store a supply of water and food. During a pandemic, it will be important to have extra supplies on hand if you can't get to a store or if stores are out of supplies. This can be useful in other types of emergencies as well, such as power outages and natural disasters.

2. Have any nonprescription drugs and other supplies on hand, including pain relievers, stomach remedies, cough and cold medicines, and fluids with electrolytes. For family members with chronic conditions, make certain that your pharmacy will be able to supply your medications.

3. Talk with family members and loved ones about how they would be cared for if they got sick or what will be needed to care for them at home.

4. Develop a way to quarantine at home, and have a plan for isolating someone who is suspected of infection or who is infected but who will not be hospitalized.

Limiting the spread of infection and preventing infection:

1. Teach children to wash hands frequently.
2. Teach children to cover coughs and sneezes with tissues, and be sure to model that behavior.

3. Teach children to stay away from others as much as possible if they are sick. Stay home from work and school if sick.

These strategies should be practiced and taught regardless of whether there is a pandemic happening in real time, simply because this strategy works best at preventing disease transmission if it's already habit before the virus reaches your community.

Glossary

#

20/80 rule: A general rule in infectious disease transmission that 1 in 5 people spreads infections within a population and controls most disease transmission events.

A

ACE2 receptor: A protein found on the surface of cells in the respiratory system, gastrointestinal tract, circulatory system, kidneys, and eyes. The receptor is the target of SARS-CoV-2, which uses the receptor as a doorway as it initiates the infection process.

Acute Respiratory Distress Syndrome: Also simply known as ARDS. The National Heart, Lung, and Blood Institute emphasizes that ARDS can occur as a result of injury, infection, or other conditions. Severe COVID-19 has resulted in ARDS for some patients.

Adaptive immune system: Immunity not present at birth that develops over time as a result of exposure to pathogens.

Adenine: A nucleic acid and one of the four constituent base compounds—building blocks—of DNA and RNA, and as such is one of the major molecules of life (see guanine, cytosine, thymine and uracil). Adenine is the letter "A" in the alphabet of life.

Adenovirus: A family of about 40 DNA viruses known to cause human infections, including the common cold. A deactivated chimpanzee adenovirus is being used in a vaccine developed at University of Oxford in England.

Aerosol transmission: Spread of disease carried via respiratory droplets transferred into the air from a cough, sneeze, or even talking or singing.

Alveolus (plural: alveoli): Tiny air sacs in the lungs where the gases oxygen and carbon dioxide are exchanged.

Anosmia: Loss of the sense of smell.

Antibodies: A complex family of proteins that plays a specific role in the adaptive immune response.

Antibody cocktail: Lab-created monoclonal antibodies based on potent natural antibodies that have been selected for their robust activity.

Antibody testing: Tests that identify whether antibodies specific to a particular infectious agent are present in a person's blood.

Antigenic shift: A change in the surface proteins of a virus that renders it unfamiliar to the human immune system, making it highly infectious, and has potential to become a pandemic.

Antivirals: Medications that interfere with the replication of viruses.

Asymptomatic: Lack of disease symptoms in a person who nonetheless is the carrier of an infectious agent.

B

Bacille Calmette-Guérin (BCG): A 100-year-old vaccine for tuberculosis that is being studied for effectiveness against COVID-19.

Binding antibodies: Antibodies that latch onto a pathogen.

B lymphocytes: Key components, of the adaptive immune system. These cells are a type of white blood cell, also known as B cells. They can form memories of previous infections, enabling a more rapid response when the infection is encountered in the future.

Budding: The process by which a virion replicates itself and emerges from a cell to seek out and infect other cells.

C

Capsid: A protein shell that protects the genetic material inside a virus.

Centers for Disease Control and Prevention (CDC): An agency of the U.S. government tasked with public health.

Chemokines: Proteins released by immune cells that attract other immune cells to the site of an injury or infection. (see cytokines).

Close contact: A person who has been within 6 feet or less of an infected individual for more than 10 minutes.

Common cold: Highly contagious upper respiratory infection caused by any one of many different kinds of viruses. There are four coronaviruses that cause the common cold. They are identified by letters and numbers: 229E, NL63, OC43, and HKU1.

Community spread: Characterized by individuals who become sick with a viral infection without knowing of any contact with someone who is ill. When individuals can't easily identify possible contacts, a viral infection is said to be spreading widely in a population.

Comorbidities: Underlying medical conditions that can complicate the progress of a newly acquired illness. *See also* Pre-existing conditions.

Complement cascade: A series of sequential activities that mark pathogens for destruction by other immune cells.

Congregate settings: Places or situations where people gather together in large groups, such as schools, summer camps, or places of worship.

Consolidation: Fluid in lung spaces that should be filled with air.

Contact tracing: The process of identifying and contacting persons who have been in close contact with a person confirmed to have an infectious disease.

Convalescent plasma: A straw-colored liquid portion of blood drawn from donors who have recovered from an infectious disease.

Coronavirus: A member of the virus family Coronaviridae, which infects a wide range of animals, including mammals such as bats. Seven strains of coronavirus are known to infect humans.

Cough hygiene: The practice of covering your mouth when you cough to limit the spread of airborne viruses.

COVID-19: The pandemic disease initiated by a coronavirus that emerged in late 2019.

Cytokines: Proteins that trigger inflammation in response to disease or injury. They include interferons (alpha, beta, and gamma), the interleukins, the tumor necrosis factor family, the chemokine family, and growth factors, which are secreted by certain cells of the immune system.

Cytokine storm: An extreme innate immune release of cytokines that can be harmful or even fatal.

Cytosine: A nucleic acid and one of the four constituent base compounds—building blocks—of DNA and RNA.

D

Deoxyribonucleic acid (DNA): The spiraling master molecule of life that contains the genetic code for all higher forms of life. This includes animals, plants, bacteria, archaea, and protists. DNA is in each cell and determines when and which life-sustaining proteins to make.

Dexamethasone: A corticosteroid drug used to reduce inflammation and tamp down the body's immune response. Doctors have had success with it treating some patients with advanced COVID-19.

Diagnostic testing: Any of several types of tests that can identify the presence of disease.

Disease burden: An estimate of the proportion of a population that is affected by a disease.

DNA vaccine: These vaccines protect against disease when an engineered plasmid—loop of DNA—bearing the code for specific viral proteins—antigens—is injected. The body's cells then produce the antigen, which is detected as a foreign sequence prompting a protective immune response and a "memory" of the sequence to develop.

Droplet: A small drop, such as a particle of moisture, discharged from the mouth during coughing, sneezing, or speaking. Droplets can contain viral particles and become airborne, which can transmit infections when others inhale them.

E

Efficient nosocomial infectious agent: A pathogen that spreads in healthcare facilities.

Endemic disease: A disease that has a constant or typical prevalence in a community.

Enveloped viruses: Viruses that have a fatty overcoat that surrounds the capsid.

Epidemic: A disease that affects a large number of people in a community; in the case of an infectious disease, sustained transmission is an epidemic hallmark.

Epidemiological data: Data related to how and in whom a disease spreads.

Essential occupations: Jobs that are defined as being vital to the well-being of a community, such as grocery workers, healthcare workers, and transportation, among others.

F

False-negative test result: A test result that shows a patient to be negative for viral infection when in fact the patient is infected with the virus. False positive is the opposite. Test result reads positive, but patient is infection-free.

Flattening the epidemic curve: A biostatistics term that means stopping new infections from developing and thereby reducing the overall number of cases.

G

Gene: The basic fundamental unit of heredity. Genes are on chromosomes and are made up of either DNA (higher organisms and certain viruses) or RNA (viruses).

Genomic vaccines: Vaccines composed of genetic sequences from DNA or RNA.

Genus: With respect to viruses, the category of the coronavirus as either an alpha- or a betacoronavirus, which

is determined by its specific molecular characteristics.

Granules: Chemical compounds produced by immune cells that defend against or identify invasive microbes.

Granulocytes: Immune cells that secrete granules to destroy invading microbes.

Guanine: A nucleic acid and one of the four constituent base compounds—building blocks—of DNA and RNA, and as such is one of the major molecules of life.

H

Hand hygiene: The practice of using frequent, thorough hand-washing to prevent the spread of diseases.

Herd immunity: Also called community immunity, which occurs when enough people in a community are immune to an infectious disease making its spread unlikely. Herd immunity is achieved through vaccination.

Histamine: A chemical produced by granulocytes that triggers inflammation in response to an injury or antigen.

Hydroxychloroquine: An antimalarial drug that is also used in treating autoimmune disorders.

Hyperendemic disease: A disease that has a high prevalence within a community or population.

Hypochlorite: A chemical produced by immune cells that kills invading microbes.

Hypoxia: Low oxygen levels in the blood.

I

Immune response: The immune system's reaction to infection, toxins, or transplanted organs

Immune senescence: The decreased response to infection related to the aging of the immune system.

Immune system: The network of cells and organs that protects and heals the body from infection, injury, and dysfunction.

Immunoglobulin: Any of the five proteins that make up human antibodies: IgM, IgG, IgA, IgE, and IgD.

Immunologists: Scientists and physicians who specialize in studying the immune system.

Incidence: The number of new cases of a disease within a specific population during a set time period.

Incubation period: The time from initial exposure to an infectious disease to the appearance of symptoms that indicate a person has been infected.

Inflammation: An immune response that triggers a set of physical and chemical reactions focused toward eliminating the threat, removing damaged tissue, and healing the affected area. Sometimes uncontrolled inflammation becomes the source of disease.

Influenza: A viral respiratory illness that occurs seasonally due to strains of influenza virus from the family Orthomyxoviridae.

Innate immune system: Protective barriers, such as the skin, as well as immune cells, and secretions present at birth that protect the body from infection.

Intensive care unit (ICU): A hospital department that gives continual monitoring and high-level care to extremely sick patients.

International Committee on Taxonomy of Viruses (ICTV): An international organization created in 1966 to classify viruses and maintain a universal virus taxonomy.

K

Kawasaki disease: An inflammation of the blood vessels that most often affects young children.

L

Leukocytes: Any of a number of white blood cells that fight disease and repair damaged tissues.

Llama antibodies: Potent antibodies isolated from llamas, which are under study as a potential treatment for COVID-19.

Long haulers: Also known as "long COVID," refers to a wide range of disparate symptoms that persist long after the evidence of SARS-CoV-2 has cleared.

Lymphocytes: White blood cells found in the lymph tissue that are important in immunity.

M

Macrophages: Large white blood cells that have the task of destroying pathogens by phagocytosis.

Memory B cell: A form of B cell that retains a long-term memory of pathogens encountered in the past.

MERS: A coronavirus disease related to COVID-19; the name is an acronym meaning Middle Eastern Respiratory Syndrome.

Messenger RNA: A single strand of RNA that directly corresponds to the instructions encoded in a sequence of DNA. That "transcript" is read by a ribosome in a cell to produce a protein.

Messenger RNA vaccine: A new type of vaccine that protects against infectious diseases. With just a single strand of mRNA, the vaccine teaches our cells to make a specific protein that triggers an immune response: the production of antibodies. If exposed to the actual virus antibodies specific to it can destroy it. mRNA vaccines are up to 95% efficacious.

Monoclonal antibodies: Laboratory-made antibodies that are used therapeutically in "antibody cocktails" to treat mild to moderate COVID-19. Monoclonal antibodies are also used to treat cancer, arthritis, and multiple sclerosis, among other conditions.

Multigenerational household: A household that is made up of more than two generations of related people—e.g., children, parents, and grandparents all living together.

Multisystem inflammatory syndrome in children (MIS-C): A rare, newly identified condition associated with COVID-19 infection in children that causes inflammation of the heart, lungs, kidneys, eyes, and brain.

Mutation: Changes that occur in genetic information.

N

Naïve B cells: B cells that have just emerged from the bone marrow and have not yet encountered a pathogen.

Neutralizing antibodies: Antibodies that make a pathogen incapable of replicating and continuing the infection.

Neutrophils: Highly abundant and mobile but short-lived white blood cells that secrete primary and secondary granules.

Non-pharmaceutical intervention: A public health effort that seeks to alter people's behavior with the goal of interrupting the chain of virus transmission in large groups of people.

O

Obligate parasite: An organism or other entity, such as a virus, that is entirely dependent on the living cells of its host.

Outbreak: A greater-than-expected increase of a disease in a population.

P

Pandemic: An outbreak of infectious disease that spreads to multiple geographic areas worldwide.

Pandemic forecasting: A proposed system of surveillance to identify infectious diseases with pandemic potential when they first emerge, with the goal of preventing pandemics.

Pandemic planning: Development of a strategy that anticipates the public health, medical, societal, and national security concerns that can arise during a pandemic.

Pathogenic: Causing disease.

Pathogen-associated molecular patterns (PAMPs): A set of general characteristics that the innate system uses to identify invasive microbes.

Pediatric inflammatory multisystem syndrome (PIMS-TS): An alternate name for multisystem inflammatory syndrome in children (MIS-C), used in the U.K.

Phagocytosis: The process of engulfing and destroying pathogenic infiltrators.

Plasma cell: A specific form of B cell that produce antibodies.

Polymerase chain reaction (PCR): A laboratory technique used routinely to identify sequences of DNA.

Precursor T lymphocytes: Developing T cells that have emerged from the bone marrow; these migrate to the thymus gland to finish their development.

Pre-existing conditions: Health issues that are already affecting an individual prior to becoming infected with a disease such as COVID-19. *See also* Comorbidities.

Prefusion: In virology, the shape of a spike protein before it latches onto the receptor that allows it to invade the cell.

Presymptomatic: This means infection has occurred and viral shedding—replication of the virus in cells—is taking place. Symptoms are not yet evident, but disease ultimately develops.

Proximate cause: The most immediate factor leading to an outcome.

Public Health Emergency of International Concern (PHEIC): A formal declaration by the WHO to highlight an extraordinary public health event that poses a risk to other countries.

R

R0: Pronounced R naught, which means in epidemiology the "basic reproductive number" of a contagious disease. Or, the average number of additional cases that directly result from one person bringing it into a community. An R0 of 2 means one person is likely to infect two others.

Rapid antigen tests: Tests that identify viral proteins (antigens); they can produce results within minutes and are designed to detect a current infection.

Remdesivir: An antiviral drug, originally developed as a potential treatment for hepatitis C, but used in a number of viral infections. It has been given an emergency authorization by the FDA for use in COVID-19 treatment. The WHO cautions that patients hospitalized with COVID-19 should not be given remdesivir.

Respiratory droplets: Tiny fluid particles that are suspended in exhaled air or expelled by coughing and sneezing. These particles can carry microbial pathogens, which are transmitted from one person to another.

Risk factor: A specific condition or situation that increases a person's risk of disease or poor disease outcomes.

Ribonucleic acid (RNA): A macromolecule that is the storehouse for hereditary information in RNA viruses. In humans, there are multiple forms of RNA with a variety of specific functions (see mRNA and Ribosomal RNA).

Ribosome (also Ribosomal RNA): The so-called "work benches" of cells where proteins are made based on instructions from mRNA. Ribosomes are also known as ribosomal RNA.

S

SARS: A highly infectious disease related to COVID-19; the name is an acronym meaning Severe Acute Respiratory Syndrome.

SARS-CoV-2: The newly identified coronavirus that causes COVID-19.

Secondary transmission: The transmission of the virus to others by an index patient, who may (or may not be) asymptomatic.

Self-quarantine: The practice of voluntarily restricting oneself to one's home and avoiding all contact with other people for a two-week period to prevent spreading an infection.

Signs and symptoms: Indicators of the presence of disease. Signs are measurable or observable indicators (fever, rash) while symptoms are subjective (fatigue, pain).

Silent spreaders: Healthy-seeming individuals who nonetheless carry a high viral load and contribute significantly to the spread of disease.

Single-stranded RNA viruses: Viruses such as SARS-CoV-2 that encode their genetic information in a single strand of RNA.

Social distancing: The practice of staying at least 6 feet away from other people to reduce the potential for virus transmission.

Specimen: Tissue or fluids collected for examination and diagnostic testing.

Spike proteins: Proteins protruding from the surface of coronaviruses. In electron microscope images, these spikes impart a crown-like, or corona-like appearance, which provides the basis of name. Coronaviruses use their spikes to initiate infection. The spikes have been targeted by most developers of SARS-CoV-2 vaccines.

Stem cells: Undifferentiated cells that have the capacity to develop into any type of cell needed.

Strategic National Stockpile: A group of large caches of emergency equipment maintained in secret locations throughout the United States.

Superspreaders: Individuals who disproportionately transmit an infection to multiple people.

Superspreader events: A documentable single event that promotes the spread of an infectious disease to large numbers of people.

T

Thymic involution: A condition in older adults in which thymus gland tissue has been replaced by fat, such that the person no longer makes new T cells in the thymus.

Thymine: A nucleic acid and one of the four constituent base compounds—building blocks—of DNA, and as such is one of the major molecules of life. Thymine occurs only in DNA, not RNA.

Thymus gland: A small gland behind the sternum that houses maturing T cells.

T lymphocytes: White blood cells also known as T cells. They are members of the adaptive immune system and fight invasive infectious agents, including viruses, and also play a role in targeting cancer cells. There are multiple types of T cells.

Triple reassortment virus: A virus such as H1N1 influenza that has genes from three different sources. In the case of H1N1, the virus had swine, bird, and human flu genes.

U

Uracil: A nucleic acid and one of the four constituent base compounds—building blocks—of life. Uracil occurs only in RNA, and as such is one of the major molecules of life

V

Vaccine: Injection of a substance relative to a specific pathogen, triggering an immune response. Administered in a minuscule dose. The aim is to prevent future infections by that pathogen.

Vaccine hesitancy movement: A belief system based on misinformation that advocates shunning vaccination. The main tenet of "anti-vaxxers" is that vaccines are dangerous to health.

Viral load: The amount of virus in the body.

Virion: The entire microbial entity composed of genes, capsid, and, if present, fatty envelope.

Virus: A submicroscopic infectious agent that requires living cells of a host to replicate and survive.

W

Wet markets: A marketplace composed of stalls that sells fresh meat, vegetables, and other perishable goods.

World Health Organization (WHO): The global agency, part of the United Nations, responsible for global public health.

Z

Zoonotic infections: Infectious agents caused by animal pathogens that have jumped the species barrier to infect people.

Index